Gut Microbiome

Repair Your Mouth Microbes to Improve Gut Health

(The Scientifically Proven Way to Restore Your Gut Health and Achieve Permanent)

Stephen Korte

Published By **Kate Sanders**

Stephen Korte

Gut Microbiome: Repair Your Mouth Microbes to Improve Gut Health (The Scientifically Proven Way to Restore Your Gut Health and Achieve Permanent)

ISBN   978-1-9994163-2-4

Legal & Disclaimer

Table Of Contents

Chapter 1: What Is Gut Health?

There is not any unmarried definition or specific profile of a 'wholesome' micro biome, and 'gut health' is a nebulous term without formal definition4, 15–17. Anecdotally, it likely encompasses the proper digestion, absorption, and synthesis of vitamins in a digestive tract that is populated with a diverse micro biome able to adapting to stressors, defensive in competition to pathogens, and appearing talents that advantage the host. Ideally, the interactions many of the host's healthy eating plan and physical interest behavior promote the boom of useful bacteria and proliferation of healthful intestinal cells and proteins that hold the integrity of the intestinal lining as a primary line of immune protection within the direction of pathogens. In flip, the bacteria synthesize nutrients that modify host metabolism and immune function in beneficial strategies. Dysbiosis is every other nebulous time period, although it's miles regularly implemented in intestine micro biome literature. Its most crucial definition is truly a microbial profile this is altered compared to a manipulate or healthful employer four, 18, 19. Researchers have diagnosed a few potentially beneficial bacteria that produce useful compounds and modulate the intestinal immune tool as well as opportunistically pathogenic bacteria that might play a function in ailment development and contamination. However, the presence of opportunistic pathogens does no longer suggest an infection, and actually they play an critical feature in coaching our immune system. Rather, it's miles the relative abundance of these micro organism that may cause—or correlate with—tremendous pathologies. It is theorized that effective microbes can also moreover moreover modify immune and inflammatory techniques via interacting with T-cells and receptors of the innate immune tool, ensuing in each pro- and anti-inflammatory cascades20–22. A vital guiding principle inside the concept of dysbiosis and illness postulates that dysbiosis

2

motives progressed intestinal permeability, permitting inflammatory or toxic contents to break out the lumen and enter the bloodstream and immune tissue beneath the intestinal cells23,24. Various varieties of dysbiosis had been located in some of ailment states, however presently, no causative hyperlink has been set up 25,26. Recent technological upgrades have shed some moderate on infection-related microbial styles which encompass the dearth of useful microbes, the enrichment of pathogenic microbes, a loss of taxonomic variety (low species richness and/or uneven distribution), and a lack of genetic (practical) diversity18,19. These changes have all been labeled as "dysbiosis."

METHODS OF IDENTIFYING BACTERIAL SPECIES AND STUDYING THE BIOME

Microbial Nomenclature

There are 3 most crucial domain names of lifestyles, all of which can be discovered in the human intestine: Eukarya (which encompass plant life, animals, and fungi), Archaea, and Bacteria.27 Eukaryotic cells encompass a nucleus and specialized structures, and often coexist to shape multicellular organisms. Yeasts and protists (parasites) are examples of eukaryotic cells that stay in our intestine, and our very private intestinal cells are also eukaryotic. Bacteria and Archaea are plenty a great deal much less complicated, current as single cells that lack a nucleus (prokaryotes). Archaea are extremophile prokaryotes which have fine in recent times been differentiated from micro organism, and little is idea approximately their feature in the gut. Bacteria are single-celled organisms that can be characterised through the usage of their anatomy (physical form) and body shape (capabilities). We prepare bacteria in businesses called taxa based totally on their diploma of genetic similarity. Viruses and bacteriophages (viruses that infect bacteria) aren't alive, but they will be positioned within the gut and can have vast impacts on each human and bacterial fitness.

4

While we do not need to memorize the taxonomy of the intestine microbiome to recognise its characteristic in human body shape, an understanding of the corporation of bacterial species is useful while decoding literature. The characterization of the human gut microbiome to this point consists of 12 phyla, which can be equal to comparing vertebrates and invertebrates6. The Human Microbiome Project has recognized twelve phyla in the human gut, but ninety% of the bacteria in the digestive tract come from simply 4 groups: Bacteroidetes, Firmicutes, Actinobacteria, and Proteobacteria1. These massive companies comprise numerous genera, which might be equal to the extent at which we group collectively puppies, wolves, and jackals. We can prepare genera into extra intently associated companies of species and sooner or later subspecies. This is critical to maintain in thoughts due to the reality the sports and potential health results of micro organism are subspecies (strain)-precise 28,29. A 'species' of micro organism is described by means of way of way of a immoderate degree of structural and beneficial similarity, however it isn't the same definition that we use to describe a species of lizards or birds30. At this element, it's miles the excellent word to be had, so we use it to differentiate between members of a genus just like we differentiate among puppies and jackals. A greater unique differentiation takes area on the amount of the stress, or subspecies, which may be likened to differentiating amongst dogs and wolves. Within a single species, a few traces are familiar additions to probiotic nutritional supplements at the same time as others are unlucky harbingers of gastrointestinal diseases. As we discover and categorize new organisms, the taxonomic tree changes and grows, which leads mockingly to more statistics further to complexity and confusion31.

Early research counseled that people might be classified into enterotypes based absolutely on the ratios of the number one phyla inside the gut (and if this sounds familiar, it is lots just like the concept of somato sorts to explain body sorts)32. Early on, a excessive ratio of Firmicutes to Bacteroidetes changed into related to the development of weight troubles, type 2 diabetes, and bowel illnesses. However, this is as improper as claiming that all vertebrates are responsible for contributing to ozone pollutants, and later systematic analyses did not help the concept 24,33. The lines of species inside those huge organizations can also have numerous consequences on gut and metabolic health, rendering the idea of an obesogenic phylum absolutely moot on the same time as including an splendid layer of complexity to analyzing interactions among those microbes and their surroundings.

Taxonomic Diversity: Who's There?

We often seek advice from the 'range' of the intestine microbiome as a function that may be indicative of fitness or disease, however this time period has one-of-a-type meanings. Diversity normally refers back to the richness (the quantity of species positioned) and evenness (the relative abundance or proportions of species in a population) of a sample34. However, a few studies most effective record indices of variety that encompass abundance, this is any other time period for richness. Richness and evenness are stricken by pattern length, sequencing intensity, and pattern processing, because the hazard for figuring out lower-abundance microbes will boom with massive sample duration and deeper sequencing, but human mistakes sooner or later of processing can reduce the accuracy of the data. These definitions of variety can be taken into consideration taxonomic considering they recognition on the individuals of the populace, however exclude the capability competencies and sports carried out with the aid of the microbes.

Researchers use quite some techniques to represent the intestine microbiome with the resource of using measuring the abundance and ratios of detectable microbes 35–37.

They try this with the aid of looking some or all of the genetic cloth of the microbiome, however of direction, the most correct strategies are also the most pricey and lots less frequently used. One common approach, referred to as 16S rRNA sequencing, uses one particular bacterial gene to understand bacteria and indicate variations at the genus and sometimes species diploma. This is frequently used in the literature, but has large obstacles as it ignores super microbes, fails to offer the important stress-unique data, and relies on curated databases to suit the genetic barcode and effectively end up aware about the samples. This method 16s rRNA records cannot imply which micro organism might be probably beneficial or dangerous, and therefore regularly outcomes in faulty conclusions approximately microbes as causative elements in fitness or illness. However, it's far useful when evaluating populations or looking at changes in a population over the years. More correct and high-priced strategies for figuring out all microbes with greater choice are referred to as 'shotgun sequencing' strategies, in which all genetic cloth is used (in region of absolutely one gene, as with 16S rRNA). This permits for identity at the species and stress degree, similarly to the inclusion of different microbes. Unlike the 16S approach, this offers notion as to the capability pathogenicity of the microbiome. Importantly, these strategies are especially sensitive, so you can regularly choose out microbes that can have enormously low abundance, but despite the fact that probably play an essential purposeful function in the intestine.

Microbes are often grouped into 'operational taxonomic devices,' or OTU's, based mostly on genetic similarity. Given that the behaviors of microbes variety on the sub-species degree, characterizing the gut microbiome with the reason to apply some correlation to health or infection arguably calls for assessment with clean decision. The kind of evaluation used after pattern collection can decide whether or not modifications may be observed38. For instance, if the assessment measures alternate on the genus degree on my own, and there are equal species fluctuations in more than one genera, the relative abundances can also appear strong regardless of variations on the pressure diploma resulting in differing useful outcomes. Fortunately, this capture 22 situation may be addressed with the useful useful resource of different way of microbiome studies. More superior strategies can pick out not pleasant lines (in a few times), but all the genetic cloth available to decide the general functionality of the microbiome. This is critical to unraveling the association many of the microbial populace, capability, and health of the host, as a one genus frequently includes many functionally first-rate species34.

Examining the variety inner one pattern is called alpha-variety, on the equal time as comparing the variations or similarities in range amongst two samples is called beta-range 35,36. Researchers may diploma richness and evenness of the stool pattern of a bodily active individual and join a quantitative charge indicating the shape of the sample. They should likely additionally quantify the alpha-form of a sedentary man or woman, then evaluate those rankings of range to determine how bodily hobby can also have an impact on the humans' gut microbiota. Alternatively, in an instance of beta-variety, they will proper away evaluate the populations of the microbes in the energetic and sedentary individuals, quantifying the distinction between the two (frequently known as dissimilarity). If their stool samples regarded notably similar, the beta-range might be low (now not very multiple).

Functional Diversity: What Can They Do?

Researchers can have a have a look at what genes (recipes for proteins) are gift in the microbiome, what genes are being expressed (the recipes being made) and what metabolites or "placed up-biotics" are gathering due to microbial metabolism39.

These strategies offer critical data approximately the useful capability and activities of the intestine. It is predicted that there are approximately one hundred,000 terabytes truely worth of bacterial DNA by myself, with even extra saved within the different microbes of the microbiome34. To complicate topics similarly, microbial gene expression is constantly converting, as are the products of microbial metabolism, making the microbiome a transferring target for practical assessment. New technology are advancing the sector, but they're first of all prohibitively pricey. Many research are limited to series of taxonomic information and now not the use of a perception into the ability sensible modifications that would rise up unbiased of adjustments inside the microbial population. In reality, some studies have confirmed that beneficial adjustments can rise up without a measurable alternate in diversity, and additionally, microbial populations that seem particular are functionally similar40. This phenomenon, called realistic convergence, has been decided even as evaluating micro

13

biomes of humans with weight issues and lean humans in unique international locations. While the microbial communities differed, they shared comparable functionality, indicating that a few organisms exhibit practical redundancy which can prevent the lack of function that might arise because of species loss. Reduced practical range has been established in people with weight troubles, and this marker may additionally function greater useful and clinically-relevant statistics than taxonomic versions.

Chapter 2: Biogeography Of The Gut Microbiome

The digestive tract is more or less 15 toes lengthy from mouth to anus, and consists of the mouth, pharynx, esophagus, belly, small and big intestines, rectum, and anus41,forty two. The accent organs encompass the liver, gallbladder, pancreas, and salivary glands. It now not great performs an vital function in the digestion and absorption of our meals, but moreover incorporates an envisioned 70% of our immune tissue and cells. The autonomic worried device regulates the specialized enteric anxious gadget of the digestive tract for the most thing, notwithstanding the fact that the enteric nervous device can act independently. Neuromodulatory chemical substances which incorporates peptides, hormones, and neurotransmitters are produced through cells in the digestive tract itself in addition to nerves from the sympathetic (combat or flight) and parasympathetic (relaxation and digest) branches of the autonomic frightened system. Most sympathetic signaling is despatched along splanchnic nerves on the equal time because the vagus nerve, which includes approximately seventy five% of parasympathetic tone, gives the parasympathetic innervation for the digestive tract. These indicators control the wavelike contractions that circulate food along, the secretion of digestive enzymes, and the contraction and rest of sphincter muscle companies that manage passage of digestive contents for the duration of—and out of—the digestive tract.

The variability of pH, anatomy, and oxygen and nutrient availability alongside the human GI tract provide a whole lot of microhabitats exerting selective strain at the inhabitant microbes2,27,forty 3. Thus, the distribution of the microbiome is quite heterogeneous, giving upward push to exceptional bio-geography from stomach to colon and lumen to mucosa. Because most microbiome studies make use of fecal samples as a surrogate for the microbial network of the whole GI tract, it is no surprise that researchers have to take some liberty in extrapolating their findings to apply to the whole microbiome. Fecal samples offer a fairly accurate common example of the colonic microbiome, but important data are frequently overlooked, leaving gaps in our contemporary understanding44. Fecal samples are clearly substantially specific from real biopsies, and individual versions are greater incredible whilst comparing biopsies in desire to fecal samples. While fecal samples usually generally tend to show extra biodiversity because they may be a difficult estimation of all microbes in the colon, only biopsies can illustrate net website online-precise variations in the microbiome along the duration of the tract or within the lumen rather than the mucosa. While maximum microbes can be observed in all fecal samples, the relative abundance can also range by means of internet net web page, and this feature is lost in a fecal sample. Additionally, some microbes can be over- or underneath-represented in fecal samples compared to biopsy samples because of internet website online online variability and sample processing34. This may additionally additionally occur because micro organism within the lumen range significantly along the duration of the intestine, whereas mucosal micro organism are an extended way greater sturdy. Because microbes have interaction with every other even as responding to environmental adjustments, growth of one organization can also inhibit or promote proliferation of every other enterprise corporation, so it is nearly no longer possible to decide what variable(s) may also account for net internet site online-precise versions in addition to the versions among fecal and biopsy samples26. That stated, it is viable to theorize the impact of host elements which include food regimen, physical interest, pH, oxygen degree, and nutrient availability on microbial populations alongside the duration of the GI tract.

Upper GI: Mouth, Esophagus and Stomach

The mouth, esophagus and belly make up the better gastrointestinal tract41,forty . The mouth produces an great 1-2 liters of saliva according to day! It is the website on line of chemical and mechanical digestion of our meals, and plays a minor function in immune defense as saliva is slightly antimicrobial. Mastication, or chewing, starts offevolved offevolved the gadget of breaking our meal down into smaller quantities that mix with the answer of water and digestive enzymes in our saliva. This mass is known as a meals bolus.

The esophagus is a 25 cm lengthy tube wrapped in 4 layers of muscle that artwork together to push our food bolus along and manipulate its release into our stomach forty one. The esophagus includes sphincters, or round muscular tissues, to control the get admission to and exit of food. If the decrease sphincter's feature is compromised, this may result in acid reflux disease illness as gastric juices from the belly can backflow into the esophagus. The characteristic of the esophagus also can be impacted by way of manner of a hernia, food hypersensitive reaction, or perhaps damage from swallowing too huge a bit of meals.

The belly is a reservoir that can stretch from 50mL to 1 or 2L in quantity, and it is a exquisite net net page of chemical digestion 41,forty five. It secretes 1-3 liters of gastric juices constant with day and continues an impressively acidic pH of about 1-2. However, the mucosa of the stomach is blanketed by using the usage of mucus secreted by means of way of specialized cells located in gastric glands. The stomach is likewise an initial line of protection in competition to capability pathogens due to the acidic contents which can be considerably antimicrobial. However, as we are able to cover later, some microbes do flourish in the stomach in spite of the antagonistic surroundings. While little or no absorption takes region inside the belly, it churns meals for 1-4 hours, mixing it with digestive enzymes. Chief cells secrete gastric lipase to break down fat as well as pepsinogen, that is cleaved to its energetic shape, pepsin, with the beneficial useful resource of hydrochloric acid. Parietal cells secrete hydrochloric acid and intrinsic element that is required for later absorption of B12. Release of these secretions is regulated via acetylcholine, histamine, gastrin, and somatostatin which is probably produced in each the stomach and small gut. Gastrin, somatostatin and histamine all paintings collectively to growth the acidity of the stomach, even as somatostatin inhibits those strategies to save you immoderate acidity. Even earlier than we start eating a meal, our senses initiate the cephalic segment of digestion, in which hydrochloric acid and pepsinogen are released in steerage of ingesting food. During the subsequent gastric section, stomach distension (stretching), and the presence of protein further stimulate the secretion of those gastric juices. Like the esophagus, the stomach additionally incorporates sphincters, and it controls the release of meals (chyme) into the duodenum, or the primary segment of the small intestine.

The intestinal section begins offevolved offevolved in response to the presence of stomach contents getting into the small gut; in assessment to the preceding stimulatory ranges, this final segment inhibits gastric motility via the release of somatostatin.

Gastric juices inside the stomach are enormously acidic, so bacterial boom and variety are restrained in the stomach27,40 3. Microbes dwelling in the ones regions ought to be aero-tolerant (able to live to inform the tale inside the presence of oxygen) and able to resist acidity; the ones requirements limit the form of the microbiome in those areas in huge element to facultative anaerobes (microbes that would make ATP without or with oxygen) that live within the direction of the epithelial cells. Many pathogenic micro organism will now not live on transit thru the stomach, this is to our advantage. Some beneficial micro organism, like Lactobacilli, can resist the acidic surroundings, or perhaps some pathogenic bacteria live proper right here as nicely. H. Pylori is one instance of a dangerous microbe associated with stomach ulcers, but it usually exists at incredibly low stages incapable of causing any damage46.

Lower GI: Small and Large Intestines

The lower GI tract is made up of about 15 toes of fleshy tubing: 10 toes of small gut and five toes of big intestine, folded notably to in shape into the stomach cavity41,40 . They are the principle website online of digestion and absorption in the body, in spite of the fact that each section can be damaged down into segments and abilities that play brilliant capabilities in the method. The whole lower GI tract is surrounded with the aid of way of layers of clean muscle referred to as the muscularis externa, which settlement to push meals alongside. The middle of the intestinal tube is known as the lumen. This is the hole space of the intestines through which digested meals movements, like water thru a hose. Between the lumen and the smooth muscle lie numerous layers of absorptive and immune cells. Technically, the lining of the digestive tract is a mucous membrane, as it's miles composed of a monolayer of mucus-protected absorptive epithelial cells supported through manner of connective tissue. This is referred to as the intestine mucosa: the bodily, bacterial, and biochemical elements of the intestines which all function collectively as a primary shape of immune safety 6,41. The bodily elements encompass the intestinal epithelium, or intestinal cells, which can be blanketed by way of the usage of one (inside the small intestine) or (inside the massive gut) thick mucus layers (one inhabited via micro organism and a deeper layer that ought to be freed from bacteria), as well as the micro organism that inhabit the intestine. Beneath the intestinal cells lies the lamina propria, a supportive connective tissue rich in immune cells. The proximity of the microbiota to the lamina propria and multitude of immune cells and receptors gives possibilities for bidirectional verbal exchange during the lifespan. Interestingly, the mucosa is considered outside to the frame, and in keeping with exceptional external surfaces, it performs an critical position in immune safety. Enzymes, antibodies, and immune cells all play an crucial characteristic in stopping illness as properly. Therefore, the intestines now not handiest function the number one website of digestion and nutrient absorption, but additionally due to the reality the first line of protection towards infectious sellers carried within the meals we consume.

Small Intestine

The shape of the small gut is specialised to maximize its ground location and contact with ingested food, as it's far the number one internet web site of digestion and absorption of nutrients41,40 two. It is crafted from 3 sections: the duodenum, this is related to the belly; the center section known as the jejunum; and the 0.33 segment this is the ileum. It joins the large intestine at a place called the cecum, but a sphincter referred to as the ileocecal valve keeps a barrier among the small and big intestine to save you backflow of digestive contents and bacteria.

This sphincter performs an essential feature in transit time by way of using controlling go with the flow of digestive contents into the big intestine in reaction to strain from food (chyme) accomplishing the latter cease of the ileum.

The whole of the small gut is packed into the belly hole space in round folds known as the folds of Kerckring 41. The internal lining of the small gut is bunched into finger-like projections referred to as villi, and the spaces between the villi are referred to as crypts. The villi are blanketed with tiny hair-like projections called microvilli. These microvilli are regularly referred to as the 'brush-border', and they're related to digestive enzymes referred to as brush-border enzymes. The crypts are home to stem cells that allow you emigrate up the villi as they mature into enterocytes, which are the specialized absorptive cells of the intestine.

The small gut is so amazingly adaptive that as a lot as 50% of it can be out of place before its beneficial capacity is affected, and people many folds boom its absorptive functionality with the useful resource of 600 times what it is probably as a at once tube.

Food movements via the small intestine due to layers of easy muscle generating wavelike contractions; that is referred to as peristalsis, and typically resembles squeezing toothpaste via a tube forty one The small intestine also plays segmentation to mix the chyme with digestive juices; those contractions are quick, oscillating segmental contractions that occur even as the peristaltic contractions waft the foodstuffs alongside. These contractions are regulated thru the enteric concerned device of the digestive tract that is in turn regulated via the autonomic stressful system. These contractions are initiated in response to the stimulus of meals stretching a phase of the gut. As digested food (chyme) moves from the stomach to the duo-denum, the hormone gastrin works together with pacemaker cells within the gut to reason contractions approximately each 10 mins until the meals bolus has reached the give up of the small intestine some three-five hours later. Even whilst the small gut is empty, the migrating motor cortex (MMC) propagates persisted, susceptible contractions approximately each 1.Five-2.Five hours to rid the lumen of any residual waste merchandise.

The small intestine produces digestive enzymes even as stimulating and receiving secretions from accessory organs 41. When food moves from the stomach to the duodenum, specialized cells inside the belly and duodenum release the hormones gastrin, secretin and cholecystokinin (CCK) in reaction to the physical stimulus of stretching similarly to the presence of acids and fats. These hormones modify gastric hydrochloric acid production, pancreatic bicarbonate and digestive enzyme secretion, gallbladder contraction for bile launch, gastric motility, gastric emptying, intestinal motility, and insulin secretion. Together, they growth churning of chyme within the stomach but save you immoderate emptying into the duodenum which needs to be cautiously buffered to manipulate pH upon arrival of the acidic chyme They concurrently loosen up the ileocecal valve, permitting the ones digestive contents to pass into the large gut and stimulate intestinal motility ordinary to move antique digestive contents out and make room for the newly-ingested meals. Meanwhile, brush-border enzymes of the small gut art work to break macronutrients into their smallest monomers for absorption (a topic a terrific way to be protected in more intensity later). As meals enters the jejunum and ileum, other hormones which include gastric inhibitory peptide (GIP), peptide YY, substance P, and glucagon-like-peptides (GLP) inhibit the sports of the belly and pancreas, lighten up intestinal contractility, and boom insulin release and blood go with the waft to the intestines to maximise the absorption and garage of vitamins. The ileum is the number one website of bile reabsorption for move decrease back to the liver; this system, celled enterohepatic bile circulate, takes vicinity six to eight times in line with day. Bile acids are able to influencing circulating levels of cholesterol in addition to the microbiota, so this manner truly performs a feature within the development of hypercholesterolemia and can additionally effect the chance of colorectal most cancers. At the terminal give up of the ileum, the ileocecal valve controls passage of chyme from the small to the large gut in which the manner of enzymatic digestion ceases and little absorption occurs.

The small intestine is the precept internet site on-line of nutrient absorption and is cut up into three sections, each with precise bacterial profiles 14,27,forty seven. The duodenum sits closest to the belly, so it keeps a greater acidic pH which limits bacterial proliferation in addition to the stomach. Here, bacterial numbers and variety are low, with Streptococcus and Lactobacilli predominating. The middle section of the small gut is called the jejunum, and due to the fact it's far much less acidic, bacterial numbers are more than that of the duodenum27,40 three. The ileum is the section of the small intestine that feeds into the cecum and big intestine. It is the maximum populous and numerous phase of the small intestine. Numbers of micro organism in the ones sections of the small intestine are to 4 times extra than that of the stomach and duodenum, and outstanding genera which incorporates Bacteroides and Bifidobacteria can thrive right here. The cecum is a massive pouch at the base of the ascending colon, and a fantastic net website online of bacterial boom as foodstuffs can pool right here and provide a wealthy supply of vitamins for the bacteria.

Chapter 3: Large Intestine

Due to sizable versions in capability, the anatomy of the massive gut is pretty one-of-a-kind from the small intestine41, forty two. Unlike the multitudinous folds of Kerckring, the massive gut is folded into just 3 quantities: the ascending, transverse, and descending colon—the latter of which results in an S-original known as the sigmoid colon. The sigmoid colon terminates on the rectum, which controls the exit of feces thru the outside sphincter; that is beneath voluntary control (maximum of the time). The large gut doesn't require good sized ground location, so it doesn't incorporate massive villi or microvilli, even though crypts in the huge intestine are in spite of the truth that gift and serve the equal characteristic as those in the small gut. Goblet cells produce big mucus, which gives upward push to the thick bi-layer of mucus masking the intestinal cells. The big intestine additionally performs contractions, referred to as haustrations, which preserve chyme in area for absorption of water and electrolytes similarly to exposure to the few colonic secretions (potassium and bicarbonate). The large intestine additionally plays propulsion, or longer contractions in numerous regions of the big intestine, and mass moves, in which huge quantities of the massive intestine settlement concurrently. Unlike propulsion, which could flow into chyme in either course, mass actions bypass chyme toward the rectum wherein defecation can take place to result in expulsion of feces. The massive intestine performs an essential feature in fluid and electrolyte balance as it absorbs those from the feces.

The massive intestine is domestic to a diverse populace of with the aid of using and huge anaerobic bacteria who feast in huge element at the nutritional carbohydrates indigestible through manner of the usage of humans27,40 3. The huge intestine, or colon, is the primary net internet page of bacterial fermentation and macronutrient metabolism, the products of which encompass gases (which consist of methane), short-chain fatty acids (which includes butyrate), neurotransmitters, amino acids, and indoles 48. Limited quantities of nutrients which include biotin and nutrients K are produced by way of the use of a few micro organism as well. Numbers of micro organism within the big gut are about ten instances greater than the ones of the belly and duodenum, and up to 2.5 instances more than the ones of the jejunum and ileum. Here, many beneficial microbes soak up residence, at the side of the butyrate producers associated with cardio-respiratory health and fiber intake. The better-most layer of mucous shielding the colonic cells serves as a safe haven and nutrient supply for some microbes that metabolize the available carbohydrates in the mucus. Thus, the luminal and mucosal populations of microbes range inside the large intestine as well2.

Poop

Feces, stool, or poop—we produce about 3 to eight oz.. Consistent with day over the path of one or some rest room visits41,forty nine. It can inform us quite plenty about our food plan, hydration repute, and health. Most people have more than 3 bowel movements in step with week, and some have 3 everyday with day (every of which is probably considered internal a normal range). Stool is normally approximately 75% water, even though this will variety based totally on healthy eating plan, hydration, and contamination. The very last 25% consists widely speakme of stupid micro organism and indigestible fiber, along with some undigested fats and ldl ldl ldl cholesterol, minerals, and mobile proteins. As stated previously, bile is produced inside the liver to assist in the digestion of fat. Feces is normally brown due to the presence of bile and bilirubin. The fragrance of stool and gas is due to the goods of bacterial metabolism of protein and fibers, together with indole, methane, and hydrogen sulfide. Drinking enough water and assembly dietary fiber dreams with a mixture of soluble and insoluble fiber each help the manufacturing of satisfactory bowel moves.

Feces can be evaluated using the Bristol Stool Chart, which charges stool consistency on a scale of one-7, with 1 correlating with constipation (small and tough, like rabbit pellets) and 7 correlating with diarrhea (absolutely liquid)40 9. Stool ought to otherwise be rated as a 3-4: sausage-formed, robust, quite smooth or a chunk lumpy, and passing with minimum straining. It need to be a coloration of brown; green, yellow, or black stool may advocate the presence of an infection or poorly-digested food41. Green stool is associated with diarrhea and may be a sign that food has moved thru your GI tract too speedy for micro organism to behave on it (as a result the lack of bilirubin-associated brown). White or clay-colored feces also can suggest low bile formation. Yellow, black, or extremely good purple stool may also additionally want to suggest severe fitness troubles which consist of an inflammatory bowel illness or intestinal bleeding. However, all the above moreover can be resulting from food coloring, glaringly-taking region food pigments, and tremendous dietary supplements or drug treatments. It is crucial to talk your rest room conduct collectively with your health practitioner in case you experience weird bowel moves to rule out the possibility of any digestive problems.

WHAT THE RESEARCH REALLY SAYS ABOUT THE GUT MICROBIOME

The intestine microbiome includes about a hundred trillion microorganisms that play important roles within the entirety from the metabolism of nutrients and manufacturing of nutrients to skeletal muscle metabolism and probably even cognitive characteristic.

There are not any standardized profiles of dysbiosis or a wholesome microbiome. "Dysbiosis" is a nebulous term that refers actually to a microbial profile that is altered in assessment to a manage or fitness institution.

Assessment of microbial variety is based on taxonomic measurements and famous the relative abundance and ratio of the microbes present in the intestine.

Measurement of the genes microbes private and the metabolites they produce offers vital facts about the realistic capacity and sports activities of the microbiome.

Colonization of the microbiome happens extensively talking in some unspecified time in the future of the primary few years of existence and is stimulated in massive part by means of using shipping and feeding techniques.

The distribution of microbes present along the gastrointestinal tract varies based truely on the variations in pH, anatomy, oxygen, and nutrient availability, with the most vital populace of microbes dwelling within the big intestine.

The number one and accent organs of the gastrointestinal tract play essential roles in digestion and absorption, in addition to immune characteristic.

The stomach homes restricted numbers and biodiversity of microbes however plays an critical characteristic in pathogen protection and the manner of digestion.

The small gut is the primary net internet web page of macronutrient and micronutrient digestion and absorption, pushed in massive detail through the release of pancreatic enzymes that further destroy down carbohydrates, proteins, and fats.

The massive intestine performs an important feature in fluid and electrolyte stability and harbors most of our intestine microbiota, which can be able to metabolizing vitamins that get away previous digestion, yielding lots of metabolites.

Stool composition tells us plenty approximately weight loss program, hydration reputation, and health reputation. The Bristol Stool Scale is a useful tool to evaluate stool consistency and may be used to help display gastrointestinal health.

DIETS AND THE MICROBIOME: FOODS AND FADS

Many factors effect an character's microbiome, which includes geographic place, start method, breastfeeding, age, gender, drug use, diet, and physical interest stages. Physical interest and dietary behavior appear to be the most elements interior our manipulate, every possibly explaining an anticipated 20% of the versions amongst individual microbiomes eleven,50. However, as illustrated in a few intervention studies, individual responses to workout, supplementation, and nutritional modifications can also furthermore range, and a few won't respond the least bit 40 4,fifty one,fifty . Some studies have verified that biomes with more variety are extra resistant to diet plan-caused modifications, at the same time as age and insufficient fiber consumption can also bunt the effective correlation between workout and microbial range. Even so, there are clean correlations amongst dietary conduct and the intestine microbiome which have been illustrated in every large-scale epidemiologic research and quick-term interventions.

To date, no unmarried dietary sample has emerged as the "accurate" preference to help the intestine microbiome, but the synthesis of records from observational studies and randomized manage trials in each people and animals have elucidated smooth traits. Dietary patterns that embody masses of quit end result, veggies, complete grains, and legumes provide masses of microbe-accessible carbohydrates, and certain foods which incorporates espresso and walnuts are related to progressed tiers of sure useful taxa 40 four,fifty three–seventy six. A high-carbohydrate, excessive-fiber weight loss program is related to a more various microbiome that consists of bacteria capable of fermenting fiber to quick-chain fatty acids useful to the gut. A high-fats, excessive-protein healthy dietweight-reduction plan is associated with a much a good deal less severa microbiome that consists of micro organism which degrade the mucous layer of the gut and launch compounds implicated within the pathogenesis of gastrointestinal ailments which incorporates colorectal most cancers. Dietary adjustments can reason fast, short fluctuations in a few bacterial species. A transfer from a Westernized, immoderate-fats diet plan to a low-fats, fiber-wealthy weight-reduction plan can produce measurable, reproducible adjustments within the microbiome profile inside 24 hours seventy two.

ENERGY BALANCE AND METABOLIC FLEXIBILITY

Although the electricity saved in nutritional fibers can not be released by using way of the use of human digestive techniques, the SCFA made from fermentation via the use of intestinal microbes can account for up to 10% of basal electricity necessities sixty six. This is called energy harvesting, and it's miles one theorized motive of the interindividual variability of predisposition to weight gain unexplained via electricity balance equations sixty six. Compared to regular rodents (colonized at starting), germ-free rodents (lacking a intestine microbiome) are proof towards weight advantage seventy seven. This may be due to versions in AMP-activated protein kinase (AMPK), which acts as an energy gauge and could increase mitochondrial fatty-acid oxidation. Multiple studies and opinions report germ-unfastened mice enjoy accelerated AMPK hobby resulting in mitochondrial biogenesis and oxidative functionality. Other research the usage of germ-unfastened mice showed a discount in each fatty acid oxidation and synthesis, which may additionally suggest an ordinary discount in energy flux (extra electricity ingested and extra energy expended). Fat oxidation and synthesis also may be regulated with the aid of the usage of enzymes which growth in liver cells after intestine colonization. One observe in healthy guys illustrated a sizable form of strength harvesting functionality, from 0-4kcal consistent with gram of ingested resistant maltodextrin that equated to an additional zero-200kcal of absorbable electricity after fermentation to SCFA available to human cells 78. Research has verified that the ones SCFA can bind to entero-endocrine cells inside the gut which adjust energy homeostasis. Certain receptors for those fatty acids are increased in subcutaneous fats of mice fed a immoderate-fat weight loss plan, and acetate and propionate have been connected to expanded adipogenesis, inhibited lipolysis, and decreased complete-body electricity expenditure in rodents. However, it need to be referred to that in some times supplementation of sure fibers called prebiotics prompted prolonged resting strength expenditure and insulin sensitivity and a decrease in fatty acid synthesis in mice, which contradicts the idea that fiber is a capacity purpose of expanded adipogenesis. Butyrate, as an instance, is a SCFA made from fiber fermentation commonly enriched within the stool of bodily-active humans. It has been confirmed to growth insulin sensitivity and energy expenditure in mice, hard the perception that fiber fermentation plays a causative function in weight benefit.

Individuals with weight issues were established to expose off lower stages of microbial and useful range, however better degrees of genes and microbes associated with energy harvesting in addition to enrichment of SCFA inside the stool 23,24,33,forty,44,50,70,seventy one,79–80 4. Lower functional variety is associated with better tiers of systemic irritation and the pathogenesis of metabolic dysregulation similarly to other chronic illnesses of the gastrointestinal tract and periphery. Studies in mice have established that colonization with micro organism from a genetically-changed mouse with obesity to a germ-unfastened lean mouse resulted in weight problems and insulin resistance with out a alternate in meals intake 77. The relevance to human beings, however, is restrained, as it's miles no longer feasible to remove the human microbiota, or maybe the software program of powerful antibiotics that appreciably reduce microbial numbers have not introduced about weight loss in humans 85. Similarly, fecal transplants from lean donors have now not been verified to modify body weight or metabolic markers in people with weight issues 86. Calorie intake seems to regulate microbial range, even though the relationship is dubious, as each more and insufficient caloric intake were related to reductions in range in a few cases 87. These findings mean a relationship amongst electricity balance, metabolic fitness, and the microbiome, though the causality and direction of this dating is still unclear.

While the link amongst weight problems and the risk of kind 2 diabetes has prolonged been installation, the microbiome is growing as an critical player inside the improvement of metabolic diseases. Metabolic endotoxemia, or chronically extended tiers of LPS which do now not reap ranges of a systemic contamination which embody sepsis however also can purpose an inflammatory response, has been implicated inside the pathogenesis of metabolic sickness 23,fifty eight,79,80. Inflammation is normally an acute, controlled approach which arises from the producing of chemical substances via the usage of immune cells in response to a stressor, which consist of workout, damage, or infection forty . These chemical materials serve to spark off all important cells of the immune system to remove the damaging substance and start the healing method. Inflammation is a everyday, wholesome response vital to immune protection, workout diversifications, and the overall protection of homeostasis. However, continual infection is associated with metabolic sickness, autoimmune troubles, and numerous gastrointestinal maladies. The problem be counted of infection has a long way an excessive amount of breadth and depth to cover inner this e-book, however it clarifies the connection many of the microbiome and metabolic illness.

Skeletal muscle is taken into consideration one among the biggest metabolically lively tissues within the frame, and in healthy humans it responds rapidly to adjustments in fuel availability (i.E., carbohydrates in place of fats)forty . Diabetes, weight troubles, and

Westernized diets are associated with notable skeletal muscle metabolism characterized thru impaired glucose managing, insulin resistance, and incomplete fats oxidation 23,forty four,fifty 8,66,eighty two,eighty 3,88–ninety. Individuals with weight troubles or kind 2 diabetes had been tested to showcase expanded degrees of LPS, the bacteria that release it, and the immune receptor to which it binds 91. Feeding studies in humans have illustrated that excessive-fat food can also moreover prompt publish-prandial elevations of LPS 90 . Skeletal muscle and fat cells precise immune machine receptors that can be activated with the aid of lipopolysaccharide (LPS) 60,ninety,ninety one. Activation of those immune receptors effects within the manufacturing of inflammatory lipid metabolites, everyday distribution of fats saved in skeletal muscle cells, and chemical messengers that result in continual, low-grade inflammation.

Chapter 4: Carbohydrates

Digestible carbohydrates may be labeled as complicated or easy based on their shape. Simple carbohydrates are made up of one (monosaccharide) or (disaccharide) rings of carbon, hydrogen, and oxygen, and those can be strung collectively to shape complicated (oligosaccharide or polysaccharide) carbohydrates forty two. Glucose, fructose, and galactose are the monosaccharides that make up all outstanding carbohydrates. The commonplace smooth sugars sucrose and lactose are located in desk sugar and milk, respectively. They're crafted from a aggregate of the monosaccharides glucose, fructose, and galactose. Fruits are immoderate in every fructose and glucose. Glycogen is the garage form of glucose, or blood sugar, in animals. Starch is the garage form of glucose in plants, and the number one complicated digestible carbohydrate in our healthy dietweight-reduction plan. It may be determined in large quantities in grains and root greens.

Chemical and mechanical digestion of carbohydrate starts in the mouth through the actions of chewing and the enzyme salivary amylase, which breaks down starch[41,40] . Not all and sundry produce salivary amylase, however it's miles of little effect because the enzyme is deactivated thru way of the acidity of belly acid. Therefore, carbohydrate digestion ceases within the belly and resumes inside the small gut. There, the digestive enzymes amylase, sucrase, lactase, and maltase damage the starch, sucrose, lactose, and maltose into the monosaccharides glucose, fructose, and galactose. Individuals with lactose intolerance do not produce lactase, so lactose isn't always damaged down correctly and as an opportunity the gut micro organism metabolize it within the massive gut, main to signs collectively with gasoline. Fibers along side cellulose contain chemical bonds that can not be damaged through the use of human digestive enzymes, so they're metabolized as an alternative by using the usage of intestine micro organism which could purpose the producing of gasoline which include methane and hydrogen, or short-chain fatty acids together with acetate, propionate, and butyrate.

Monosaccharides input the enterocyte via protein channels embedded inside the mobile membrane42. Glucose and galactose every input the intestinal cell thru SGLT-1; the way requires each energy and the presence of sodium. Fructose, however, enters via way of GLUT5; at the identical time as this manner does not require strength or sodium, it's miles depending on the attention of fructose inside the intestinal cellular. Thus, if there may be an abundance of fructose already in the mobile, the the rest is probably trapped inside the lumen. This can entice water into the lumen and bring about gastric dissatisfied and diarrhea. Once within the enterocyte, all 3 monosaccharides diffuse into the bloodstream through GLUT-2. Just just like the passive get right of entry to of fructose into the intestinal cellular, the get admission to of monosaccharides into the bloodstream is a passive tool based totally upon the eye in the bloodstream. These key additives of carbohydrate digestion and absorption dictate the vitamins pointers round exercise. By ingesting the proper kinds of carbohydrate in the right recognition and on the proper charge, viable beautify absorption and save you gastric disappointed all through exercise to sell better overall performance.

Resistant starch is a shape of starch awesome from the kind that without hassle breaks proper all the way down to glucose ninety three. There are five sorts of resistant starch which may be placed in unprocessed grains and legumes, green bananas, and raw potatoes, however those starches additionally can be long-hooked up at some stage in cooking and processing. Manufacturers can produce some sorts of resistant starch, and others shape as a result of heating and cooling starchy meals, together with potatoes and rice. There is some evidence that repeated heating and cooling of these materials will increase the resistant starch content cloth cloth, and this in flip should have a notable impact on regulating blood glucose and feeding beneficial bacteria inside the gut51,90 three.

Studies in each animals and people have illustrated that dietary patterns which incorporates complex carbohydrate, resistant starch, and fiber from whole grains, end result, legumes, and veggies are actually correlated with microbial variety and human fitness 6,forty four,51,66,sixty nine,seventy 3–seventy five,90 3–95. Replacing delicate grains with whole grains has been proven to enhance urge for food manipulate, blood glucose law, and growth numbers of SCFA-producing bacteria. Low-carbohydrate and diffused-carbohydrate diets which might be low in fiber had been verified to lessen numbers of useful Bifidobacteria and fecal butyrate. Additionally, a immoderate-carbohydrate food plan is related to greater numbers of Prevotella, a genus of micro organism that is typically higher in exercisers in assessment to sedentary people.

Fiber

It is important to be aware that, due to the fact fiber plays such an important feature in microbial metabolism, complete grains in choice to sensitive grains need to be prioritized. Fibers are carbohydrates which is probably indigestible to people 40 ,sixty seven. Fibers are labeled by means of using their solubility, viscosity, and fermentability. Most soluble fibers are with out issues fermentable and may or may not additionally be viscous (because of this forming a gel in a liquid surroundings). Insoluble fibers are typically poorly fermentable and non-viscous, however they though play an essential characteristic in gut fitness. The insoluble dietary fibers along side cellulose, hemicelluloses, and lignin are determined in brans, cereals, legumes, vegetables, and fruits (specifically the skins). Beta-glucans, pectins, and fructans are all soluble, and encompass the maximum not unusual dietary fiber, inulin (a fructan). These are positioned in whole grain merchandise, potatoes, legumes, vegetables, and surrender quit end result as nicely. It is good to ingest a aggregate of each soluble and insoluble fiber to feed the microbiota, shape bulk in the stool, take in extra cholesterol, and ease the transit of stool41.

The fermentability of a fiber can be the maximum massive trouble in identifying its potential to have an effect at the microbiome sixty seven,68,ninety four,96. Most soluble fibers are fairly fermentable and feature the exceptional impact, increasing numbers of useful Bifidobacterium and Lactobacillus; the ones embody fructans and galacto-oligosaccharides generally found in whole grains and legumes. Fiber fermentation effects predominantly within the formation of brief-chain fatty acids with a few gases (methane and hydrogen) as well. The primary SCFA's produced are acetate, butyrate, and propionate; lactate and succinate are also produced in smaller portions. These SCFA's play important roles in urge for food regulation, intestinal barrier feature, insulin signaling, lipid metabolism, pathogen suppression, and colorectal maximum cancers protection. They might also furthermore provide up to ten% of our every day caloric requirements48! Pectin is broadly speaking fermented to acetate, which may additionally moreover have maximum cancers shielding consequences within the frame via regulating apoptosis and preventing oxidative damage to cells ninety six. Butyrate serves as a number one fuel source for intestinal cells and might furthermore exert protecting results in competition to colorectal maximum cancers. Because nutritional butyrate is absorbed via the host within the small intestine, the most effective supply of butyrate for the microbes and intestinal cells of the large intestine might be that produced via bacterial fermentation of microbe-to be had carbohydrates. Propionate is a excellent substrate for gluconeogenesis inside the liver, and today's studies have demonstrated that athletic populations residence positive micro organism that produce this SCFA in big portions in assessment to sedentary human beings. Inadequate fiber consumption has been related to thinning of the protective intestinal mucous layer and disruption of everyday microbial biogeography in rodent models 6,59,sixty three. A modern-day have a take a look at in bodybuilders positioned that the ones consuming insufficient fiber (~15g/day) exhibited tons much less microbial range than humans who've been assembly the RDA; in fact, their microbial variety become now not substantially unique from sedentary controls97. While there may be however an lousy lot to be discovered, it is easy that a excessive-fiber food plan (meeting or exceeding the RDA of 25g/day in women and 38g/day in grownup males) gives a large number of health blessings mediated largely by manner of the intestine microbiota forty one.

Classifications of Dietary Fiber

Classification EffectsTypes

Soluble   Dissolves in warmness water; absorbs water inside the GI tract

Delays gastric emptying and could boom transit time

Can decrease nutrient absorption (e.G., fat)

Aids inside the cut price of ldl ldl cholesterol

Many soluble fibers are fermentable   ß-glucans, gums, wheat dextrin, psyllium, pectin, fructans

Insoluble   Generally, does not soak up water in the GI tract

Decreases intestinal transit time

Increases fecal bulk (acts as a "broom" within the gut)   Lignin, cellulose, some hemicellulose

Fermentable Refers to fibers which can be metabolized thru way of the intestine microbiota (prebiotics)

Primary cease merchandise encompass numerous gasses and short chain fatty

May want to be restricted in human beings with IBS or one of a kind GI situations due to excessive gas manufacturing   ß-glucans, guar gum, wheat dextrin, pectin, fructans

Viscous/Gel Forming   Similar to soluble, however no longer all soluble fibers are gel forming

Increases gastric distention, delays gastric emptying, and could boom transit time

Reduces / delays nutrient absorption

Traps bile ➔ decreased micelle formation, lipid absorption, and recirculation of bile (mechanism for reducing ldl cholesterol)   ß-glucans, guar gum, psyllium, pectin

Types of Fiber and Food Sources

Type of Fiber Characteristics   Food Sources

Pectins   Mixed solubility

Fermentable

Viscous/gel forming Apples,   strawberries, raspberries, citrus quit end result, legumes, oats, and a few vegetables

Gums Soluble

Fermentable

Viscous/gel forming Legumes, oats, and barley

Cellulose   Insoluble

Non-fermentable Found in maximum plants due to its role within the plant cellular wall Legumes, nuts, wheat bran, root vegetables, peas, cruciferous greens, apples, and outdoor a part of seeds.

Hemicellulose   Mixed solubility

Mixed fermentability   Whole grain products, bran, legumes, and nuts

Fructans   Soluble

Fermentable Asparagus, garlic, onion, artichoke, chicory root, bananas, barley, and rye

ß-glucans   Soluble

Fermentable

Viscous/gel forming Primarily located in oats and barley

Resistant starches   Mixed solubility

Mixed fermentability   Unripe bananas, legumes, rice, pasta, cooked & cooled potatoes, excessive amylose corn, in part milled grain products and a few seeds

FODMAP's and Gastrointestinal Distress

Some individuals enjoy immoderate symptoms of irritable bowel syndrome or gastrointestinal misery after ingestion of sure fermentable carbohydrates called FODMAP's75,98,ninety nine. This acronym refers to "fermentable oligosaccharide, disaccharide, monosaccharide, and polyols" which include fructose, lactose, sorbitol, mannitol, fructans, galactooligosaccharides, and sugar alcohols. These carbohydrates are in reality and fermented and can also exert osmotic hobby which pulls water into the lumen of the gut. This can bring about bloating, gas, stomach pain, and diarrhea.

FODMAP's are typically determined in an entire lot of beans, give up quit result, wheat, dairy products, nuts, and every fibrous and starchy vegetables. Many humans are understandably stressed after they experience uncomfortable digestion after making nutritional changes to boom the fiber or nutrient density of their healthy eating plan with the beneficial aid of ingesting more of these 'healthful' ingredients. Unfortunately, unscrupulous practitioners and entrepreneurs regularly try to monetize this phenomenon via claiming that it is a signal of 'awful intestine fitness,' while in fact is it virtually the quit result of live organisms generating power and through the usage of-products.

The Low-FODMAP Diet changed into in recent times evolved via Monash University as an intervention for human beings with Irritable Bowel Syndrome (IBS) ninety eight–a hundred. A low-FODMAP weight-reduction plan isn't intended for prolonged-term adherence as a loss of soluble dietary fiber could have terrible results on the microbiome (which includes reductions in Bifidobacteria), but it's far a beneficial tool to strategically put off and re-introduce food to decide their impact on one's gastric issues. It is usually encouraged to comply with a low-FODMAP diet for two weeks in advance than introducing unique food or corporations of FODMAP-containing elements in a systematic way even as watching symptoms of gastric misery alongside side fuel, bloating, and extraordinary bowel moves. This approach need to be pur-sued with steerage from a practitioner who has been knowledgeable or certified thru the Monash Low-FODMAP software application.

Fermentable Oligo-, Di-, and Monosaccharides and Polyols

Poly & Oligosaccharides   Disaccharides
        Monosaccharides   Polyols   (Sugar Alcohols)

Inulin

Galacto- (GOS)

Fructo- (FOS)

Isomalto- (IMO)   Lactose   Fructose
        Sorbitol Mannitol

Malabsorption is giant in humans because of lack of digestive enzyme   Malabsorption might also additionally rise up due to lactase enzyme deficiency Absorbed slowly inside the small gut, especially while ingested by myself or in more of glucose   Absorbed slowly   inside   the   small   intestine; malabsorption isn't always unusual

Pass thru small intestine and are rapidly fermented in the large gut Attracts water to the huge intestine where it is also fermented   Pulls water into small intestine and/or passes to big gut wherein it's fermented Pull water into small gut and/or pass to massive intestine wherein they're fermented

Beans, cabbage, onions, chicory root, legumes   Dairy products (in diverse amounts)   Apples, pears, artichoke, asparagus, honey, fruit juices   Pears,   apples,   pitted culmination, cauliflower, mushrooms, weight loss plan ingredients/ beverages

FAT

Fats can be labeled as saturated or unsaturated; maximum saturated fat are of animal beginning and stay solid at room temperature, whilst many unsaturated fat are of plant beginning and stay liquid at room temperature one zero one. These can be further divided into monounsaturated and polyunsaturated fats, the latter of which includes omega-3 and omega-6 fatty acids. Omega-9 fatty acids can be monounsaturated or polyunsaturated and are placed in loads of plant oils. Unsaturated fat play vital roles in inflammatory techniques and are largely cardioprotective.

Fat digestion starts in the mouth, wherein lingual lipase starts offevolved offevolved to break down nutritional triglycerides into mono- and diglycerides41,40 . Unlike salivary amylase, lingual lipase isn't always deactivated by means of the use of stomach acid. As fat enters the duodenum, the gallbladder responds via releasing stored bile (produced via the liver) and the pancreas produces its personal version of lipase. The bile acids surround lipid debris to create an emulsification, or combination of tiny lipid globules suspended in the aqueous environment. This allows the lipase enzymes to break down the triglycerides greater efficaciously; without this emulsification approach, the triglycerides might also need to accumulate just like the manner oil bureaucracy globules in vinegar. The breakdown of triglycerides, called lipolysis, cleaves the fatty acids from their glycerol backbone. The length of the fatty acid chain determines its absorptive route. Short-chain fatty acids can freely diffuse thru the enterocyte, getting into skip right away. Longer chain fatty acids have to be transported into the enterocyte in which they are re-associated with a glycerol backbone and packaged as a lipoprotein referred to as a chylomicron. The chylomicron enters lymphatic movement earlier than entering into the bloodstream in which it starts its journey to the liver, shelling out lipids to tissues along the manner. Very little fat reaches the massive intestine, and notwithstanding the truth that some microbes own lipases that could cleave fatty acids from their glycerol spine, their interactions with glycerol are restricted and unsure. Free fatty acids aren't carried out as an strength deliver with the aid of the microbiota, but they will modify the populace of microbes no longer without delay via immune receptor binding, pH law, and stimulating the producing of bile48.

A immoderate-fat eating regimen (normally >40% power from fat) has been linked to low-grade infection termed 'metabolic endotoxemia', wherein portions of bacterial cell partitions (endotoxins) escape the gut and set off an immune response that has been implicated in insulin resistance and obesity 23,24,forty four,seventy nine,eighty,ninety two. High-fat diets appear to lessen the range of the microbiome, and especially reduce numbers of Bifidobacteria and every so often Lactobacilli, on the equal time as growing specific strains of Firmicutes that have been related to the improvement of weight troubles 23,40 4,fifty 4,66,seventy two. Eight weeks of a calorie-limited (30% deficit), ketogenic-style (four% power from carbohydrates) added about a decrease in Bifidobacterium and butyrate concentrations 102. Similar results have been seen after 4 weeks of a mild-carbohydrate weight-reduction plan (35% calories from carbohydrates) or a ketogenic-style weight loss plan compared to a weight loss program with ~50% energy from carbohydrates. A small widespread sort of studies in frame and staying electricity athletes have illustrated a negative correlation among fats consumption and Bifidobacteria or ordinary range in fiber-bad diets 97,103. This will be because of a loss of fiber which ends up in a reduction in Bifidobacteria and/ or an growth in protein intake that is associated with prolonged numbers of Bacteroides. Because epidemiological research can handiest illustrate establishments, and intervention studies do now not preserve fiber consistent among controls, it's miles dubious whether or not or not a weight loss plan excessive in fats and fiber might have the same outcomes due to the fact the excessive-fats, low-fiber diets studied thus far. Recent rodent research have illustrated that the principle culprit may be the insufficient fiber consumption, as each excessive- and coffee-fats fiber-terrible diets exerted comparable results on the microbiota. The loss of Bifidobacteria also can purpose reduced stages of butyrate, a SCFA utilized by intestinal cells for electricity. Bacteroides are identified mucin degraders, and in mice, a reduction in the defensive mucous layer has been illustrated because of fiber deficiency. Together, the ones factors can purpose improved intestinal permeability and expanded levels of circulating endotoxins which encompass lipopolysaccharides (LPS). These changes had been shown in humans after a unmarried immoderate-fats meal project, and LPS appears to be chronically extended in a few people with weight troubles, as well as rodent models of weight issues 1,23,forty four,fifty eight,90,ninety two.

Few research have examined the effect of specific macronutrient kinds at the microbiome, and presently there may be little proof that nutritional fat kind affects the human microbiome in a excellent manner compared to the consequences of carbohydrate intake. Diets excessive in saturated animal fat appear to preferentially boom numbers of mucin-degrading bacteria, markers of infection, intestinal permeability, and now and again fats benefit in comparison to diets containing immoderate stages of unsaturated fat 23,44,60,seventy four,90 ,104,one zero five. Monounsaturated fats and omega-6 polyunsaturated seem to elicit similar results on severa beneficial bacterial traces (i.E., discount in Lactobacilli and Bifidobacteria), probable because of the reality that the ones bacteria focus on metabolizing precise plant-based totally compounds 106. Omega-three polyunsaturated fats also can lessen endotoxin concentrations after a excessive-fats meal (35% energy from fat) in comparison to saturated fats that have been established to acutely growth plasma endotoxin ranges 90 two. Additionally, omega-three supplementation has been demonstrated to briefly boom numbers of Bifidobacteria, Lactobacilli, Lachnospira, and Roseburia—all of that are useful, quick-chain fatty acid producers 106.

This isn't to mention that animal fat reason weight troubles or contamination in isolation. Rather, it illustrates the connection most of the microbiome, dietary fats, and capability for metabolic dysregulation, as adipose tissue inflammation has been identified as one feasible element inside the improvement of kind 2 diabetes 23. Based at the evidence up to now, it seems that saturated fats have a greater capacity for growing inflammatory tone at the same time as omega-3 fatty acids may also moreover confer a few advantages.

Additionally, fiber intake probable affects the microbial response to one in all a kind stages of fat intake and fatty acid composition.

Chapter 5: Protein

Proteins are crafted from amino acids and may be categorized as excessive- or low-fine primarily based totally on each their digestibility and ratio of amino acids one zero one. Of the 20 amino acids, nine are considered essential due to the fact they can't be produced through way of the human frame. A great protein includes sufficient ranges of all important amino acids to promote increase and restoration and is also effects digested. A low-awesome protein will lack adequate tiers of one or greater of these critical amino acids and can additionally be plenty less bioavailable. Some plant substances are considered 'whole' proteins because they do embody all the essential amino acids, but they may now not consist of quantities which can be adequate for the help of increase and healing if eaten in isolation. In elegant, animal proteins are considered wonderful with the aid of method of these requirements, on the equal time as plant proteins commonly lack one of the important amino acids and are less digestible. Many property of plant proteins additionally offer more fiber, a whole lot less saturated fats, and beneficial plant compounds that aren't positioned in animal proteins, and they will moreover be an lousy lot tons much less highly-priced. Soy protein does consist of all 9 crucial amino acids at the side of a number of fitness blessings.

While acidity inactivates a few enzymes, it could spark off others, as is the case in protein digestion41,forty . When meals enters the stomach, hydrochloric acid cleaves the enzyme pepsinogen to its energetic form pepsin. Together, the acidic surroundings and the interest of pepsin each "untangle" dietary proteins and start to cleave the bonds between man or woman amino acids, ensuing in short polypeptides. In the small gut, greater pancreatic proteases damage the ones polypeptides into even shorter chains and in the end single amino acids. Thus, it isn't whole proteins, however amino acids and quick peptides which might be absorbed into the enterocyte. This takes place via specific transporters for single acidic, important, and independent amino acids, or PEPT1 which non-discriminately transports di- and tripeptides into the cellular. Thus, short peptides can be extra successfully absorbed. Like monosaccharides, the absorption of amino acids and peptides calls for the presence of sodium. Inside the enterocyte, maximum of these peptides are in addition broken down into unmarried amino acids which then enter motion. Amino acids that reap the massive gut may be fermented to short- or branched-chain fatty acids or gases, converted to special amino acids, or degraded to indoles and phenols which can have toxic, neuromodulatory, or carcinogenic results 48.

Few studies have examined the effects of immoderate-protein diets on the gut microbiome, and they come with confounding variables even as you don't forget that elevated protein at the identical caloric consumption calls for a lower in both fats or carbohydrates. High-protein diets have been connected to advanced frame composition and decreased urge for food, possibly in issue because of amino-acid derived compounds produced through way of intestine micro organism (i.E., GLP-1, serotonin) forty four,107. However, epidemiological research have related everyday intake of pink and processed meats to elevated risk of colorectal most cancers and inflammatory bowel illnesses thru products of amino acid fermentation 44,seventy four. Several research have proven that excessive protein intake is correlated with improved numbers of Bacteroides which produce some of the compounds associated with colorectal most cancers and atherosclerosis 44,48. The production of these compounds seems to be higher with habitual ingestion of beef compared to bird. Other research have established that the effects depend upon the specific kind of protein; for example, animal proteins in famous may additionally additionally growth or decrease numbers of Bifidobacteria and Bacteroides, and whey protein can also boom stages of every Bifidobacteria and Lactobacilli on the same time as reducing numbers of Bacteroides 71,104,108. Some taxa also can ferment amino acids, ensuing inside the manufacturing of SCFA which can be of gain, but moreover unfavorable compounds together with amines, phenols, sulphides and thiols that have been related to colorectal cancers and colitis 48. The manufacturing of these compounds may be decreased if adequate microbe-to be had carbohydrates are provided 109.

The most relevant finding regarding protein intake and the gut microbiome can be the importance of the protein:fiber ratio, because the disparity among these nutrients also can play a characteristic in the production of in all likelihood risky compounds produced through amino acid fermentation. While one perfect ratio hasn't been determined, cutting-edge-day proof allows the advice of meeting at least the encouraged each day intake of fiber ninety seven,109.

Effects of Macronutrients, Alcohol and Caffeine at the Microbiome

Macronutrient   Effects

Carbohydrates   Complex carbohydrates, resistant starch, and fiber associated with diversity

Replacing diffused carbohydrate with complicated belongings elevates numbers of SCFA-generating bacteria

Reductions in today's or complex carbohydrate consumption associated with reduced Bifidobacteria

Inadequate fiber intake related to thinning of intestinal mucus layer, disruption of everyday biogeography, and suppressed impact of exercising on range

Lipids High-fat (>forty% kcal) diets linked to metabolic endotoxemia & reduced range

Saturated fat might also moreover acutely growth circulating LPS

Omega-three fat do not induce elevations in LPS after a excessive-fat meal and may increase numbers of beneficial micro organism

High fats intake at the rate of carbohydrate or fiber is associated with decreased range and proliferation of mucin-degrading bacteria

Proteins   High protein intake associated with improved numbers of Bacteroides, which degrade mucin & produce metabolites related to colorectal maximum cancers

Amino acid fermentation can also motive SCFA manufacturing, but might also moreover produce carcinogens

Adequate fiber consumption can also attenuate volatile results of excessive protein consumption

Alcohol & Caffeine Moderate consumption of pink wine related to greater variety in observational research

Chlorogenic acid in espresso might also additionally exert bifidogenic consequences and decorate range

MICRONUTRIENTS

The time period micronutrients refers extensively to vitamins and minerals that perform crucial functions within the human body41,forty . Vitamins may be in addition subdivided into every fat soluble (nutrients A, E, D & K) or water soluble (B-nutrients & vitamins C). Minerals are classified as important (calcium, phosphorus, sodium, potassium, chloride, magnesium, sulfur) or hint (iron, copper, zinc, selenium, iodine, chromium, fluoride, manganese, molybdenum) primarily based on the relative quantities required with the useful resource of the human body. Differences within the form and chemical composition of these micronutrients—in addition to the health recognition and functionality of the gastrointestinal tract—have an effect at the place and amounts absorbed. The routes of absorption for nutrients and minerals variety extensively, with a few requiring protein corporations to pass for the duration of the intestinal mobile and others freely diffusing into or between intestinal cells. In regularly, micronutrient absorption is inversely correlated with ingestion; in distinct phrases, absorption ranges growth at the same time as nutritional availability is low. Most nutrients and minerals may be absorbed with the aid of the usage of the usage of the small gut. Sodium, potassium, and chloride are exceptions; they'll be absorbed usually within the huge gut due to their capabilities as electrolytes and association with water. Additionally, a few vitamins, especially nutrition K and biotin, may be synthesized with the beneficial resource of the gut microbiota and subsequently absorption within the colon can get up as nicely. However, this microbial synthesis isn't concept to make contributions that extensively to the overall stages of these nutrients inside the body.

A sort of nutritional elements can effect micronutrient absorption, both enhancing and inhibiting the device forty one. For instance, fat soluble weight-reduction plan absorption can be better via manner of consumption with a meal containing fat, iron absorption may be better via diet C. Sometimes physiological elements which include age or intestinal illness will lessen the body's ability to take in nutrients. Vitamin B12 absorption requires the presence of gastric intrinsic element, which may be decreased in older human beings. Supplementation also can avoid micronutrient absorption. Excessive fiber intake can also moreover moreover disrupt intestinal absorption of many nutrients and minerals, at the identical time because the presence of wonderful minerals may moreover moreover obstruct the potential of various minerals to be absorbed because of sharing transporters or transport mechanisms. For example, excessive nutritional or supplemental intakes of zinc or iron can intervene with absorption of copper. It is essential to also factor out that medicinal drugs have the potential to impact micronutrient absorption, and over-the-counter dietary nutritional dietary supplements also can interact with medicines. Little is understood about microbiome-micronutrient interactions, but rising evidence shows that effective vitamins and minerals, which include vitamins A and D and iron, may also moreover exert have an effect on on the microbial profile thru host immune law one hundred ten. Vitamins A and D are critical to gut barrier integrity as they play a function in tight junction regulation and cell differentiation. Micronutrient deficiencies, specifically of folate and B12, may additionally exert epigenetic results during fetal improvement and young people that could additionally effect the growing microbiome.

Chapter 6: The Gut-Brain Connection

Few connections in our body form are as charming and influential because the dynamic interaction among the intestine and the brain. This economic damage is a journey into the clinical nuances of this connection, similarly to a revelation of approaches facts and harnessing it could redefine our intellectual readability, emotional stability, and regular cognitive feature.

Your Second Brain: The Enteric Nervous System

The path to records the gut-mind connection begins off evolved with the identity of the enteric worried device (ENS), moreover called the "second thoughts." The ENS is a complex network of neurons that operates independently of the valuable involved system, nestled inside the partitions of the digestive tract. As I dug deeper into the studies, I located that this'2d mind' does more than absolutely coordinate digestion; it additionally communicates bidirectional with the mind in our skulls, influencing our emotions, thoughts, or even desire-making techniques.

Neurotransmitters and the Modulation of Mood

The characteristic of neurotransmitters, the chemical messengers that allow neurons to speak with each different, has been a pivotal discovery in the take a look at of the intestine-thoughts axis. Notably, the intestine produces a massive amount of serotonin, a neurotransmitter this is usually related to temper regulation. The implications are profound: our gut fitness has an immediate effect on our emotional well-being. I speak how imbalances inside the intestine micro biome will have an effect on serotonin manufacturing, doubtlessly contributing to tension and depression.

Gut Micro biome: Neurotransmitter Designers

As we delve deeper into the gut-thoughts connection, we encounter the designers of neurotransmitters: the trillions of microorganisms that include the intestine micro biome. It becomes smooth that intestine bacteria and neurotransmitter production have a symbiotic courting (meaning that they depend upon each different for survival nearly like a natural couple). Bacterial traces play an essential role inside the synthesis of neurotransmitters, offering a unique attitude on intellectual fitness interventions that circulate past pharmaceutical techniques. In this phase, I present actionable strategies for cultivating a micro biome that promotes most exciting neurotransmitter stability.

Inflammation and Cognitive Implications

The hyperlink amongst gut fitness and brain function goes beyond neurotransmitters to encompass infection. Chronic inflammation, it's far regularly as a consequence of an imbalanced gut, has a ways-accomplishing results on cognitive skills. I look at the pathways by means of which inflammatory signs excursion from the intestine to the mind, doubtlessly contributing to cognitive decline and neurological troubles. Gut-centric interventions to reduce infection take center stage, presenting want for no longer most effective digestive health however furthermore cognitive sturdiness.

Leaky Gut Syndrome: The Doorway to Neurological Disarray

As awkward because the choice may want to possibly sound "Leaky intestine," is a condition wherein the intestinal barrier becomes compromised, allowing undesirable materials to go into the bloodstream, is gaining interest within the medical community. The effects of a leaky intestine circulate beyond digestive ache, doubtlessly influencing the neuroinflammatory cascade and contributing to neurological troubles. I speak the complicated courting between leaky intestine and situations like Alzheimer's and Parkinson's illness, emphasizing the significance of gut integrity in keeping cognitive fitness.

Real-World Strategies for Maintaining a Healthy Gut-Brain Axis

The bankruptcy concludes with sensible techniques for cultivating a resilient and harmonious intestine-mind axis as we traverse the hard landscape of the gut-thoughts connection. Each strategy, from dietary interventions that promote neurotransmitter synthesis to manner of lifestyles practices that lessen irritation and sell intestine integrity, is a step inside the route of improving your intellectual readability, emotional resilience, and cognitive prowess.

We've peeled over again the layers of the intestine-mind connection in Chapter 1 of this e-book, revealing a symbiotic courting that defies conventional knowledge. As you encompass the ones insights and placed into effect the practical techniques referred to, keep in mind that optimizing your gut health is ready unlocking the complete capability of your intellectual and emotional properly-being. Welcome to the charming international of the intestine-brain connection, wherein the affect pathways amongst your 2d and 1/3 brains hold the vital component to a existence of readability, stability, and cognitive brilliance.

Chapter 7: The Micro Biome Blueprint

As we hold to forge in advance valiantly via the enchanting landscape of intestine fitness, Chapter 2 well-known the micro biome blueprint—a microscopic global teeming with trillions of microorganisms that have an impact on the whole lot from digestion to immune characteristic. In this financial ruin, we will take a look at the complex balance that is required for a resilient micro biome and offer sensible tips for cultivating a severa network inside.

A Diverse Ecosystem Revealed via the usage of the Micro biome

First, apprehend what the micro biome is. The micro biome is an surroundings extra various than the Amazon rainforest that lives inside the gut. This community of bacteria, viruses, fungi, and different microorganisms performs a symphony of capabilities vital to our health. As we preserve I will delve in addition into the micro biome's awesome variety, emphasizing the importance of maintaining a balanced and varied composition for max remarkable well-being, retaining matters smooth, concise, and brief.

Digestive Harmony and Gut Micro biome

The position of the micro biome in digestion is the number one save you on our adventure, this is often overshadowed via its broader implications. Microbe's useful aid inside the breakdown of complicated carbohydrates, the extraction of essential nutrients, or maybe the regulation of our urge for food. I show how specific nutritional alternatives can genuinely impact microbial variety, selling efficient digestion and nutrient absorption, the usage of some realistic examples.

Probiotics and Prebiotics: Feeding the Microbial Orchestra

When it involves proactive gut health, probiotics and prebiotics are key players in nourishing the microbial symphony inside. Probiotics, which is probably beneficial micro organism positioned in fermented components and dietary dietary supplements, boom the microbiome's range and resilience. Prebiotics, as an alternative, are indigestible fibers that feed the ones beneficial microbes. I'ii display you in short the way to consist of probiotic-wealthy food like yogurt, kimchi, and sauerkraut into your each day food regimen, as well as prebiotic assets like garlic, onions, and bananas.

Fermented Foods' Gut-Healing Potential

Fermented elements act as culinary alchemists, remodeling raw factors into dietary powerhouses that supply a lift to the intestine vegetation. I guide you thru the sector of fermented delights, from the tangy enchantment of kombucha to the probiotic-wealthy allure of kefir. Practical examples and recipes are furnished, making it clean to embody the ones intestine-friendly additives into your each day routine, thereby supporting the increase of useful bacteria and fostering a resilient microbiome.

Antibiotics and the Gut Microbiome

While antibiotics are important inside the remedy of bacterial infections, their indiscriminate use can disenchanted the touchy balance of the microbiome. I shed slight at the collateral damage that antibiotics can purpose to gut fitness and provide realistic techniques for mitigating their outcomes. These practices, which variety from centered probiotic supplementation to consuming probiotic-wealthy meals in the path of and after antibiotic guides, feature a blueprint for restoring microbiome resilience.

Personalized Microbial Diversity Nutrition

Here, I'd like to emphasize vividly that your microbiome is as specific as your fingerprint. Recognizing your strong point is critical in growing a custom designed technique to intestine health. I introduce the concept of personalized nutrients based totally definitely for your microbial profile, demonstrating how specific dietary choices correspond to the dreams of your individual microbiome. Practical examples and pointers allow you to make informed alternatives which might be regular together with your intestine's particular desires.

Lifestyle Habits for a Healthy Microbiome

Aside from nutrients, way of lifestyles alternatives have a massive effect at the microbiome. I offer sensible insights into fostering a microbiome-first rate lifestyle, starting from the impact of strain on microbial balance to the gut-loving benefits of regular physical hobby. These easy changes will allow you to contain intestine fitness into your each day recurring, growing an surroundings that promotes the increase of your microbial allies.

The microbiome blueprint is your manual to cultivating range, resilience, and balance in this health lawn. With realistic examples and actionable strategies in hand, you are equipped to embark on a adventure toward a thriving microbiome and, as a give up give up result, progressed nicely-being.

Gut-Healing Nutrition: Crafting a Culinary Symphony for Digestive Harmony

The palette of gut-restoration nutrients is discovered out in this bankruptcy of the gastronomic odyssey of gut fitness—a symphony of substances that no longer only nourish the frame but moreover foster an surroundings conducive to most useful digestion and microbiome balance. This chapter is especially for the foodies right here and as this sort of culinary adventure in which every chunk has the capability to bolster your gut and enhance your number one health.

Prebiotic Power: Fueling Your Microbial Allies

The frequently-not noted electricity of prebiotics—nondigestible fibers that serve as gasoline for the beneficial microbes to your intestine—is at the coronary coronary heart of gut-healing nutrients. From the earthy crunch of asparagus to the candy indulgence of bananas, I delve into the arena of prebiotic-wealthy food. Practical examples and easy recipes are furnished to illustrate the way to without issue consist of these prebiotic treasures into your each day meals, presenting nourishment for the growth of your microbial allies.

Probiotic Wealth: Growing a Diverse Microbial Garden

Probiotics, which is probably stay useful bacteria found in fermented factors and dietary supplements, play an crucial position in cultivating a numerous and resilient microbiome. From the tang of Greek yogurt to the fizz of kombucha, I'ii gladly regale you with a sensory adventure of probiotic-rich delights. Practical examples and progressive recipes show off a manner to include those microbial allies into your food plan, enhancing your intestine health with every delicious bite.

Fiber's Crucial Function: A Digestive Symphony

Setting out on a fiber-centered dietary adventure is similar to wearing out a digestive symphony. Fiber-rich components behavior this symphony with the useful resource of encouraging everyday bowel moves, stopping constipation, and developing an surroundings that promotes intestine fitness. I recommendation which you consume more of fiber-wealthy elements like entire grains, legumes, end end result, and veggies to expose your plate right into a canvas of digestive harmony.

Anti-Inflammatory Elixirs: Turmeric, Ginger, and Other Ingredients

This segment makes a speciality of contamination, which is often a silent disruptor of gut health. I introduce the culinary international's anti inflammatory heroes, in conjunction with turmeric and ginger, highlighting their sturdy homes and realistic applications. Recipes infused with those anti-inflammatory elixirs emerge, presenting not first-rate gastronomic satisfaction but additionally a barrier closer to intestine contamination, making sure your digestive machine operates in a snug and balanced nation.

Oily Wonders with Gut-Loving Omega-three Fatty Acids

Omega-three fatty acids, which can be placed in fatty fish, flaxseeds, and walnuts, have emerged as key game enthusiasts within the gut-healing repertoire. These oily wonders no longer first-class decorate average coronary coronary heart and thoughts fitness, but additionally they have anti-inflammatory effects in the gut. Practical examples of incorporating omega-three-wealthy components into your diet plan are provided, demonstrating how those nutritional powerhouses may be effects blanketed into your culinary routine.

Gut-Healing Spices and Herbs: A Flavorful Pharmacy

In this phase, the spice cupboard is transformed proper into a flavorful pharmacy as we observe the medicinal houses of herbs and spices. Here, I take you on a short sensory journey of intestine-recovery treasures, from the digestive prowess of peppermint to the soothing consequences of chamomile. Practical examples and infusion recipes might be supplied, reworking your kitchen proper right into a haven for herbal remedies that sell digestive well being.

Fermented Delights: Creating a Probiotic Feast on Your Plate

Continuing from Chapter 2, we delve deeper into the vicinity of fermented delights, reworking your plate proper right into a probiotic feast. Practical examples and fermentation recipes are furnished to illustrate a manner to master the art work of fermentation at domestic. Each chew will become a party of intestine fitness, introducing a numerous array of probiotic lines on your microbial network, from sauerkraut to kimchi.

Imagine your plate as a canvas as you navigate the culinary symphony of intestine-recuperation nutrients in this financial ruin of the e-book with each element contributing to the masterpiece of digestive harmony. You're no longer simply nourishing your body if you have realistic examples and recipes at your fingertips; you're cultivating an environment indoors that resonates with strength, resilience, and gut fitness.

Chapter 8: Digestive Detoxification

In the look for maximum incredible gut fitness, this economic disaster lays out the framework of digestive cleansing—a method that is going past cleansing to resume and revitalize your intestine surroundings. This bankruptcy is a manual to flushing out pollutants, rejuvenating your digestive tool, and growing an surroundings that helps prolonged-time period well-being, from targeted nutritional selections to life-style practices.

Digestive Detoxification: More Than Just Cleansing

Digestive cleaning is a holistic technique to helping your frame's natural detox strategies, in preference to intense cleanses or deprivation. This phase delves into the complexities of digestive cleansing, looking at how the liver, kidneys, and digestive tract artwork together to take away pollution. Understanding this technique lays the foundation for practical techniques that art work collectively along with your body's natural detoxification mechanisms.

Hydration as a Detox Elixir: Water, Lemon, and Beyond

Water, the elixir of lifestyles, is undisputedly at the coronary coronary heart of digestive detoxing. Hydration emerges as a foundational pillar, facilitating waste and toxin elimination from the body. I delve into the transformative electricity of water, offering practical techniques for reinforcing your hydration routine. Lemon water, it is high in antioxidants, becomes a powerful first-class pal for your digestive detox adventure.

Fiber's Detox Dynamo: The Cleansing Embrace

Fiber, a normal hero inside the intestine fitness story, takes middle diploma all yet again due to the fact the detox dynamo. High-fiber meals act as natural brooms within the digestive tract, sweeping away waste and pollution. This phase illuminates realistic examples of fiber-wealthy meals, offering a avenue map for infusing your diet regime with the cleansing power of whole grains, fruits, and veggies.

Teas for Detoxification: Chamomile, Peppermint, and Dandelion

As we inspect the detoxifying houses of herbal teas, their soothing embody takes middle degree. These teas end up allies in your digestive detox adventure, from the calming effects of chamomile to the digestive prowess of peppermint. Practical examples and brewing pointers are provided that will help you include the ones detoxifying elixirs into your every day ordinary.

Liver Support: An Important Aspect of Detoxification

The liver, as a detoxification powerhouse, deserves particular interest in this segment. I talk the liver's position in processing and eliminating pollutants, in addition to realistic techniques to useful resource its feature.

From cruciferous vegetables like broccoli to antioxidant-wealthy herbs like milk thistle, we examine dietary options that growth the liver's natural detoxification abilities.

Fermented to Cruciferous Gut-Cleansing Foods

Certain components assist to cleanse the gut thru the usage of promoting toxin expulsion and fostering a wholesome microbial surroundings. We delve into the world of intestine-cleaning foods, from fermented delights to cruciferous greens that help cleansing enzymes. Practical examples and recipes are supplied to help you embody those cleaning treasures into your culinary repertoire.

Fasting and Intermittent Detox: Periodic Gut Resets

This phase specializes in intermittent fasting and detox strategies that offer your digestive gadget with relaxation and rejuvenation. There are realistic examples of intermittent fasting styles and detox protocols given, permitting you to tailor your method to your life-style and dreams. These periodic resets deliver your gut the distance it needs to regenerate and thrive.

Digestive Renewal Through Mindful Eating

Mindful consuming is going beyond nutrients to end up a cornerstone inside the digestive cleansing way, the antique pronouncing of one being what they consume has its birthplace from aware eating, in nearly all the vitamins books read and written through wonderful authors which include the fitness meetings I actually have attended, the amazing paintings of conscious ingesting has been one of the few ordinary mentions. I walk you thru the ideas of aware consuming, imparting sensible recommendation on a manner to domesticate focus of your food alternatives, eating conduct, and the signs and symptoms your body sends. Mindful ingesting is a transformative practice that promotes a stronger connection among your thoughts and your gut.

Think of this Chapter as you may a slight motion flowing thru your digestive landscape, visualize it clearing away debris, nourishing the soil, and renewing the environment inner. The artwork of digestive cleansing turns into a holistic adventure of renewal when you have realistic examples and actionable techniques at your disposal.

Stress Management Techniques: Nurturing Your Gut Amid Life's Storms

Chapter 5 of this e-book reveals an essential act within the dynamic dance of intestine fitness: stress control a topic I understand all-too-nicely as a medical doctor. Stress, an ever-present stress in present day lifestyles, has the potential to have an effect on no longer best our intellectual fitness however moreover the sensitive balance of our digestive machine. This financial catastrophe is a manual to enforcing strain control techniques that now not most effective relieve every day burdens however additionally nurture a resilient and flourishing gut.

Stress as a Disruptor: The Gut-Brain Connection Revisited

We move back to the problematic tapestry of the intestine-mind connection earlier than delving into pressure management strategies. Stress, it seems, is greater than best a highbrow state; it has a physiological impact at the intestine. Understanding this link is vital as we embark at the direction of pressure control strategies that now not best calm the thoughts but additionally promote intestine fitness.

Mindfulness Meditation: Developing Presence within the Face of Chaos

The historical exercising of mindfulness meditation is at the forefront of stress control. This method isn't about casting off pressure; as a substitute, it is about cultivating a present cognizance that modifications our courting with it. In this section, I will walk you thru mindfulness meditation practices, offering you with practical examples so that you can can help you incorporate moments of mindfulness into your every day regular, fostering a feel of calm that extends from the mind to the gut.

Techniques for Deep Breathing: Oxygenating Your Gut

The breath, a rhythmic dance many of the outdoor worldwide and your internal being, will become a effective pressure-cut price tool. In instances of pressure, deep breathing strategies which includes diaphragmatic respiration and field breathing function anchors. Practical examples and step-with the resource of-step instructions are furnished to help you harness the calming have an effect on of your breath, oxygenating not simplest your thoughts however moreover your intestine.

Progressive Muscle Relaxation: Release Tension From Head to Toe

Techniques that relieve bodily pressure gain the gut extensively, which is usually a silent repository of anxiety. In this regard, Progressive Muscle Relaxation (PMR) emerges as a treasured exercising. I stroll you thru the procedure of systematically exciting muscle businesses, offering realistic examples that allows you to assist you to launch tension not only from your shoulders, but moreover from the very middle of your digestive tool.

Yoga for Gut Health: Bringing Movement and Mindfulness Together

Yoga, an historical exercise that mixes movement and mindfulness, has developed into a complete technique to stress control. Yoga poses and sequences are designed especially to promote gut health, combining the benefits of bodily interest with the calming balm of mindfulness. Practical examples and illustrations can lead you through a yoga adventure that no longer incredible promotes flexibility and energy, but additionally a peaceful intestine environment.

Nature Therapy: The Healing Power of Nature

Nature's healing include becomes a powerful stress control device, offering solace amid the chaos of each day lifestyles. Nature treatment, furthermore known as ecotherapy, entails immersing your self in natural environments to relieve stress and enhance well-being. I offer concrete examples and techniques for incorporating nature remedy into your day by day ordinary, like, taking lengthy walks in lots less populated woods basking in nature's energy and alluring the recuperation contact of nature to soothe each your thoughts and your intestine.

Emotional Release Journaling: A Gut-Heart Connection

In this segment on journaling, the written phrase serves as a conduit for emotional launch. Chronic strain frequently harbors unstated emotions, that would take area in the gut. Journaling offers a solid vicinity for these feelings to be untangled, fostering a gut-coronary coronary coronary heart connection. The journaling method is each guided by using manner of sensible examples and activates, or without any of the above allowing you to unburden your mind at the identical time as also nurturing your intestine.

Establishing Boundaries: Protecting Your Gut Sanctuary

Boundaries are essential inside the digital age for maintaining our highbrow and intestine health. This part of the e-book delves in quick into the paintings of putting boundaries, whether or not or not with work, generation, or social responsibilities. Practical techniques are to be located supplying you with the equipment to guard your intestine sanctuary from the outside international's relentless demands, permitting it to regenerate and thrive.

These pressure-good deal strategies said are a symphony of practices, each be conscious resonating with the capability to assuage your mind and nourish your intestine. Stress manage turns into a transformative adventure with practical examples and actionable techniques—a aware try to aid your intestine in competition to existence's storms.

Fitness for Gut Health: A Symphony of Movement and Microbes

This financial ruin starts offevolved off from in which the preceding financial disaster ends as it proceeds into symphony of movement and microbes inside the rhythm of gut fitness. Fitness, it is regularly lauded for its benefits to physical well-being, furthermore has a massive impact at the intestine microbiome. This chapter makes it a factor of duty to stroll you thru the machine of creating a health routine that now not simplest nurtures your frame but moreover fosters a thriving microbial community internal.

Beyond Physical Fitness: The Gut-Exercise Connection

Before beginning a health routine, it's miles important to apprehend the complex dating the various gut and exercising. It appears that the intestine reacts dynamically to bodily hobby. In this section, we're going to observe how exercise affects the intestine microbiome, digestion, and preferred intestine health, laying the groundwork for a symbiotic courting amongst fitness and the microbial worldwide indoors.

Cardiovascular Exercise and Gut Health Pacing

Cardiovascular workout, with its rhythmic and sustained nature, emerges as an important participant in gut fitness guide. Keep your eyes on severa cardio exercise routines, from brisk on foot and walking to biking and swimming. These sports activities now not most effective enhance cardiovascular fitness but moreover contribute to a numerous and resilient gut microbiome, fostering a digestively healthy environment.

Microbial Resilience Strength Training

Strength training, commonly defined as resistance sports that target muscle development, will become a foundational issue of our health symphony. Strength training physical video games the use of body weight, unfastened weights, or resistance bands are validated. Strength training no longer simplest strengthens your muscle tissues however moreover has a extraordinary effect in your intestine microbiome, fostering a microbial network that thrives in reaction to the physical needs of resistance physical sports.

Yoga and Gut Health: Microbial Landscape Balancing

In this section, yoga, it is famend for its holistic approach to nicely-being, takes middle degree. Yoga poses and sequences are designed to sell gut health. I provide practical examples of yoga exercising routines that no longer best improve flexibility and stability, but additionally create a harmonious surroundings within the intestine. Yoga fosters a thoughts-body connection this is nurturing to the gut microbiome.

Microbial Metabolic Boost with High-Intensity Interval Training (HIIT)

High-Intensity Interval Training (HIIT), which incorporates quick bursts of excessive interest accompanied thru short periods of relaxation, has emerged as a dynamic pressure in our fitness orchestra. HIIT exercising sporting activities are proven in element, demonstrating how this form of exercising not exceptional improves metabolic fitness but furthermore stimulates microbial range and metabolic activity within the intestine, contributing to most best digestive function.

Microbial Diversity and Outdoor Exercise

In this section, nature serves as a dynamic backdrop for fitness. Hiking, going for walks, or biking outdoor now not most effective offers bodily blessings but additionally exposes you to pretty some environmental microbes. I endorse you walk thru a few practical examples of out of doors health sports activities, inviting you to take in some smooth air and display your gut microbiome to the diverse microorganisms discovered in natural settings.

Post-Workout Nutrition for Gut Health

Post-exercising vitamins performs an crucial position inside the fitness journey for intestine fitness. Practical examples of put up-workout gut-boosting meals and snacks are furnished, within the shape of emphasizing the importance of nutrient-dense components. These alternatives no longer best help with muscle restoration, but similarly they offer important nutrients that assist the gut microbiome, ensuing in an surroundings that prospers after physical hobby.

Consistency and Adaptability: The Keys to Long-Term Fitness

With a focal point on consistency and flexibility, the symphony of health for intestine health reaches a crescendo. A normal health habitual this is tailor-made in your alternatives and lifestyle turns into an essential component in long-term gut health. Following noted sensible strategies useful resource in keeping consistency and adapting your health normal to changing instances, ensuring that the symphony of movement and microbes keeps for years to come.

Here's a amusing exercise that you may strive, as you study through the pages of this financial disaster near your eyes in short and accept as true with your self as a conductor, orchestrating a symphony inside your body— envision each melody of fitness and notes of vitamins completed as ones which may be in sync with the microbial community to your gut. Fitness becomes a holistic journey that nurtures your intestine, fosters resilience, and contributes to the flourishing of your stylish fitness with realistic examples and actionable techniques.

Chapter 9: Sleep Optimization

The focal factor of this chapter is inside the quiet realm of intestine fitness, targeted at the frequently overlooked however profoundly impactful realm of sleep. This financial ruin is a step-through-step guide to coming across the secrets and strategies of sleep optimization, revealing how the excellent and duration of your sleep have a superb effect at the fitness of your gut and, via using extension, your state-of-the-art fitness.

A Bidirectional Influence on the Gut-Sleep Connection

Before delving into sleep optimization techniques, it's far essential to understand the complex dance the various intestine and sleep. The intestine-sleep connection is bidirectional, with the intestine influencing sleep first-rate and the sleep influencing gut functionality. This phase delves into the charming interplay the various intestine microbiome, circadian rhythms, and sleep tiers, laying the idea for the transformative journey of sleep optimization.

Circadian Rhythms: Sleeping in Time with Nature

Circadian rhythms, which might be internal clocks that adjust physiological techniques over a 24-hour cycle, function our guiding lights in terms of optimizing sleep. Practical examples and strategies for aligning your sleep patterns with the natural ebb and go with the float of circadian rhythms are presented. By embracing steady sleep-wake cycles and exposing yourself to herbal slight for the duration of the day, you synchronize your inner clock with nature's rhythm, promoting top of the street sleep first rate.

Sleep Hygiene: Creating a Stress-Free Sleep Environment

Creating a sleep sanctuary turns into an important element of optimizing sleep. Practical examples of sleep hygiene practices are supplied, guiding you to create a non violent slumbering environment. These techniques, which encompass limiting publicity to digital gadgets earlier than bedtime, adjusting room temperature, and making an funding in a snug mattress, pave the way for a restful and rejuvenating night's sleep.

Evening Relaxation Rituals: Unwinding the Gut and Mind

The hours earlier than bedtime end up a sacred ritual for unwinding and getting ready your belly and mind for restful sleep. Allow me to attract your attention thru a few practical examples of exciting nighttime rituals like moderate stretching, analyzing, and mindfulness exercise. By incorporating those rituals into your pre-sleep regular, you could create a smooth transition from the stresses of the day to the serenity of the night time.

Nutritional Sleep Support: The Gut-Friendly Bedtime Snack

Nutrition will become an crucial nice friend in the pursuit of maximum important sleep. The function of particular nutrients in selling relaxation and supporting a restful night time's sleep is highlighted through sensible examples of intestine-first-class bedtime snacks. From sleep-inducing herbal teas to tryptophan and magnesium-rich snacks, those options now not best nourish your intestine but additionally decorate the extremely good of your sleep.

Physical Activity and Sleep Quality: A Powerful Combination

If you are like me who revels on the concept of hearty wearing activities then you'd be pleased to realize that the approach of physical sports activities, which become previously lauded for its effect on intestine health, now takes middle level inside the realm of sleep optimization. Exercise physical activities that resource sleep great are illustrated with practical examples, demonstrating how regular physical hobby contributes to deeper and additional restorative sleep. By incorporating those carrying sports activities into your normal, you enhance each your intestine health and the high-quality of your sleep.

Stress Reduction for Better Sleep: Calming the Gut and Mind

Stress, which is mostly a nocturnal intruder, can upset the delicate balance of sleep. This a part of this monetary spoil revisits strain manage techniques designed specially for the nighttime, offering practical examples that soothe both the gut and the thoughts. These practices, which variety from guided relaxation physical video games to deep breathing techniques, help to create a non violent mental environment conducive to restful sleep.

Sleep Supplements and Aids: Gut Harmony Support

Targeted supplementation can be a treasured device in the adventure to better sleep for some people. Practical examples of sleep nutritional dietary supplements and aids are tested, together with melatonin, magnesium, and herbal extracts. Understanding the function of these nutritional nutritional supplements in promoting relaxation and improving sleep extraordinary allows you to make informed picks which can be tailored on your unique wishes and opportunities.

Equipped with actual-international examples and actionable strategies, this bankruptcy initiates the protocol for sleep optimization which turns into a transformative adventure that promotes now not only your relaxation but furthermore the health of your intestine environment.

Gut-Immune Axis Fortification: Building Resilience from Within

The starting of bankruptcy eight tells us a tale of a fortress-building tour in the realm of holistic well-being—a guide to fortifying the intestine-immune axis. This bankruptcy, in addition delves into the intimate relationship some of the gut and the immune device, revealing how gut health can reason a resilient immune response. We embark on a adventure to construct a robust safety from inside, the usage of realistic examples and actionable strategies.

The Gut-Immune Axis: A Symbiotic Partnership

Before delving into fortification strategies, it's critical to understand the symbiotic dating that exists many of the intestine and the immune device. As the body's largest immune organ, the intestine consists of a complicated network of immune cells, and the immune device is predicated on the intestine for training and steering. This segment delves into the complex dance of the gut-immune axis, laying the idea for the fortification journey.

Gut Microbiome Diversity: An Important Factor in Immune Vigilance

Microbial diversity inside the gut emerges as a key player in immune device fortification. Clarification right here is available in form of walk-thru of a few sensible examples of nutritional and way of life alternatives that promote a numerous microbiome. Incorporating some of give up give up result and veggies, as well as embracing fermented materials, all make contributions to a thriving microbial network, training the immune device to apprehend and respond to a huge kind of threats.

Prebiotics and Probiotics: Gut Immune Allies

In this section, prebiotics and probiotics, which have been formerly mentioned for his or her function in intestine health, over again take the middle degree as immune allies. Examples of prebiotic-rich meals and probiotic sources are highlighted, demonstrating how those additives improve the gut-immune axis. Prebiotics and probiotics guard the immune gadget thru offering essential vitamins for beneficial micro organism and introducing stay microorganisms.

Immune-Boosting Nutrients: Gut Defense

Nutrients derived from a numerous and nutrient-dense diet serve as armor for the intestine and immune tool. I pass over sensible examples of immune-boosting vitamins like healthy eating plan C, nutrition D, zinc, and antioxidants, emphasizing their roles in immune characteristic. You lay the muse for a resilient immune reaction for your self by the usage of manner of prioritizing a healthy eating plan wealthy in these vitamins.

Gut Integrity and Immune Defense: A Barrier of Protection

The integrity of the intestine barrier, that is regularly compromised in modern-day-day existence, is critical in immune defense. Let's in quick walk you via a few practical examples of behavior that sell intestine integrity, which include eating fiber-rich meals, heading off antibiotic overuse, and proscribing your exposure to intestine irritants. A robust gut barrier acts as a protecting guard, preserving risky substances out of the bloodstream and triggering immune responses.

Immune Hygiene Hydration: The Defense Elixir

Hydration, previously recognized for its function in digestive health, now unsurprisingly serves as a cornerstone in immune hygiene. Practical examples of staying efficaciously hydrated, with a focal point on water consumption, are endorsed. Hydration promotes mucosal immunity, making sure that the intestine mucous membranes continue to be a resilient first line of protection toward pathogens.

The Nocturnal Guard: Sleep and Immune Resilience

Sleep, which have become stated in element in a separate chapter, reappears once more as a effective fantastic pal in immune resilience. Practical examples of fostering healthful sleep behavior want to be revisited, with an emphasis at the vicinity of restorative sleep in supporting immune cell feature. By putting first rate sleep first, you decorate your immune device's capacity to find out and combat capacity threats.

Stress Management: Bringing the Immune Storm Under Control

This phase investigates the impact of strain on immune feature, a normal topic at some level within the holistic fitness adventure. The position of strain manage strategies in calming the immune typhoon is highlighted through sensible examples. These practices, starting from mindfulness meditation to deep respiration bodily games, make a contribution to immune resilience with the resource of mitigating the negative consequences of continual strain.

It ought to serve you better at the forestall of this monetary disaster to usually envision the gut-immune axis as a dynamic alliance, with each method serving as a brick in the castle of resilience. You're no longer genuinely fortifying your intestine with practical examples and actionable techniques; you're nurturing a safety device the likes of which has in no manner been visible earlier than it is prepared to face the annoying situations of the out of doors international.

Chapter 10: Hormonal Harmony For Gut Health

Chapter nine begins off evolved out as a symphony of hormonal harmony and a manual to knowledge and cultivating balance within the hormonal panorama for maximum satisfying gut health. This financial disaster delves into the dynamic interaction amongst hormones and the gut, offering sensible examples and strategies for promoting balance, electricity, and digestive properly being.

The Hormonal Orchestra: Gut Health Conductors

Before embarking at the hormonal concord journey, it's miles important to pick out out the key conductors within the hormonal orchestra. Hormones are critical regulators of many physiological processes, collectively with digestion and gut feature. This phase delves into the complicated dance of hormones inside the frame and their effect at the gut, laying the idea for the hormonal symphony.

Cortisol and Digestion: Stress Response Navigation

In this phase, cortisol, that is often associated with the pressure response, takes center degree. I stroll you through the consequences of cortisol on digestion, emphasizing its role in gut characteristic modulation. Practical examples of pressure manipulate techniques need to be revisited from preceding chapters. By reducing the terrible consequences of continual pressure, you can create an environment wherein cortisol stages are balanced, thinking of most satisfying digestive function.

Leptin and Ghrelin: Hormonal Satiety Partners

The hormones leptin and ghrelin, which adjust urge for meals and satiety, become focal elements in our investigation of hormonal harmony. Practical examples of dietary picks and manner of life conduct to resource hormone stability are furnished. These encompass consuming a nutrient-dense eating regimen, consuming often, and running closer to conscious eating, through this, you promote a harmonious dating amongst leptin and ghrelin, promoting healthy digestion and weight management.

Insulin Sensitivity: Blood Sugar Balance for Gut Wellness

Insulin, a key regulator of blood sugar, sticks out proper right here as an important conductor in the hormonal symphony for gut fitness. Practical examples of dietary and way of life alternatives that sell insulin sensitivity are stated proper right here. These strategies, which variety from ingesting fiber-wealthy meals to challenge regular physical interest, all make a contribution to strong blood sugar levels, growing an environment that promotes gut well being.

Thyroid Hormones and Metabolism: Digestive Pace Influencers

An now not probably traveller flourishes on this phase, the Thyroid hormones, which modify metabolism, have an impact on digestion and intestine functionality. I'ii in short stroll you via practical examples of the way nutrients and way of life choices can help you guide thyroid fitness. Did you understand that by means of the usage of certainly incorporating iodine-rich meals, selenium resources, and pressure control, you may assist to stability thyroid hormones and enhance the performance of digestive strategies in the intestine.

Sex Hormones: Menstruation and Gut Health

Menstrual cycles and sex hormones are critical game enthusiasts within the hormonal orchestra for women. There are practical examples of how to guide intestine health in the course of the menstrual cycle. Women can tailor their nutrients and self-care practices to beautify digestive well-being for the duration of the menstrual cycle through manner of know-how the innate hormonal fluctuations that arise at some point of menstruation, ovulation, and the luteal segment.

Serotonin and Mood Influencers inside the Gut-Brain Axis

In our investigation of hormonal harmony, the intestine-mind axis, a two-way communication device, will become a focal point. Serotonin, a neurotransmitter that affects temper and digestion, takes the spotlight. Practical examples of dietary alternatives and life-style behavior that sell serotonin manufacturing inside the intestine are provided. You create a effective feedback loop that promotes each emotional nicely-being and digestive health thru nourishing the gut-brain axis.

Hormonal Balance and Adaptogens: Nature's Harmonizers

Adaptogens, herbs, and botanicals that have been established to modulate stress responses and hormonal stability become no longer going allies in our quest for hormonal balance. Adaptogenic herbs which includes ashwagandha and rhodiola are examined in detail. By incorporating adaptogens into your everyday, you create a conducive environment for hormonal balance, selling resilience and balance inside the body.

By the save you of this financial ruin you'll have a whole health orchestra at your ft and an interplay of rhythms and melodies that compose body's stability. You're now not sincerely harmonizing your hormones even as you operate practical examples and actionable techniques; you are cultivating an surroundings wherein the intestine and the hormonal orchestra are in sync.

Gut-Driven Longevity: Nurturing Lifelong Vitality

The message of this monetary disaster is sturdiness or to area it higher, intestine-pushed sturdiness—a guide to fostering lifelong strength via the cultivation of intestine fitness—in the grand tapestry of nicely-being. This financial disaster delves into the profound courting among a thriving intestine and durability, offering practical examples and strategies for nurturing the symbiotic relationship a few of the gut and the pursuit of an extended, colorful life.

The Longevity Blueprint: Uncovering the Gut Connection

Before we embark at the direction of gut-driven durability, we should first recognize the blueprint that links the intestine to the quest for a protracted and vibrant lifestyles. The intestine, also referred to as the "second thoughts" and the "coronary coronary heart of health," will become a focus in the observe of sturdiness. In this phase, we are able to examine the scientific proof for the way a healthful intestine contributes to everyday sturdiness.

Gut Microbiome and Aging: Inside the Fountain of Youth

The gut microbiome, a severa community of microorganisms that live inside the digestive tract, is emerging as an vital aspect inside the getting older manner. There are sensible examples of dietary options and manner of existence conduct that beneficial aid a healthful gut microbiome. Such examples range from ingesting fiber-wealthy food, fermented delights, and prebiotics which promotes microbial variety, paving the way for a gut-driven fountain of young adults inside.

Inflammaging and Gut Health: Managing Time's Flames

Inflammaging, or continual and espresso-grade inflammation related to getting older, plays an essential function in our studies of intestine-pushed toughness. Practical examples of anti-inflammatory dietary and way of life alternatives are provided. By which consist of substances excessive in antioxidants, omega-3 fatty acids, and gut-soothing herbs, you can create an surroundings inside the gut that combats the inflammatory techniques associated with growing vintage.

Cellular Senescence: Gut Nutrients' Role in Renewal

Cellular senescence, the dearth of a cell's capability to divide and feature, is inextricably associated with the growing older approach. Here's a brief walk-via some actual-worldwide examples of gut-amazing vitamins that sell cell renewal or a rejuvenation of cells if you may. These meals, which range from the ones excessive in polyphenols and antioxidants to those immoderate in important nutrients and minerals, all make a contribution to the upkeep of cell strength, fostering a intestine-driven method to durability.

Gut-Brain Axis and Cognitive Aging: Mind Nourishing

The intestine-brain axis is studied on the subject of cognitive getting old, that is regularly associated with a decline in cognitive function over time. There are realistic examples of food that promote brain fitness and cognitive feature. You nourish now not simplest your intestine however moreover your mind by way of way of manner of prioritizing a food regimen rich in omega-three fatty acids, antioxidants, and thoughts-boosting vitamins—a holistic approach to promoting toughness.

Hormonal Harmony as an Orchestrator for Longevity

Hormonal balance, that is mentioned in detail in a separate financial disaster, reappears over again as a crucial problem inside the quest for toughness. Practical examples of the manner gut-satisfactory practices can help assist hormonal harmony are revisited. These examples embody eating food that balance insulin, cortisol, and intercourse hormones, via doing this, you can create an inner environment that is in sync with the rhythms of durability.

Gut Integrity: A Protective Factor Against Aging

The integrity of the intestine barrier turns into essential within the pursuit of gut-pushed durability. There are sensible examples of behavior that promote intestine integrity. By collectively with bone broth, glutamine-rich components, and restricting exposure to gut irritants, you could pork up the intestine barrier, which acts as a guard in competition to the wear and tear and tear and tear of time.

Gut-Driven Longevity Nutrition: A Culinary Symphony

In the very last movement of our journey, we are going to see sensible examples of a intestine-pushed durability weight-reduction plan—a culinary symphony that syncs up with the rhythms of a long and colorful lifestyles. From antioxidant-wealthy berries to intestine-soothing herbs and spices, every aspect gives to the concord of dietary choices that promote gut health and durability.

What thoughts section through your thoughts as you have a look at the very last of "Men's Ultimate Gut Health Hacks that Work," a symbiotic dating some of the seeds of intestine fitness and the blossoms of a protracted, colourful lifestyles. You're now not clearly extending the amount of your life with practical examples and actionable techniques; you are also nurturing the exceptional of your years, fostering a journey of electricity and properly-being.

Chapter 11: Prepare To Learn No Longer Alone

Have you ever felt like no man or woman is familiar with you or what you're going through? Welcome to a network of people who experience and think just like you. Many of the people who've picked up this eBook have lengthy gone via similar evaluations. Some days your signs may be mild; different days, it may enjoy as despite the fact that your stomach is experiencing a pounding and a half of! Those days can get us down. We might also additionally revel in lousy, tiresome, and aggravated while the signs and symptoms and symptoms and signs and symptoms regress. When those symptoms and signs and symptoms get worse, they might paintings on our tension and strain our bodies out. Does it ever look like you cannot capture damage? This is how I felt for a long time until I discovered a way to manipulate my fitness.

Gut inflammation, next signs, and contamination may additionally have an effect on quite plenty surely every person. It is especially common in a society that eats for comfort in a short-paced way of life. In this approach, the excellent of food, the shape of meals, and the portions of fatty materials ingested turn out to be a blur. Antacids are the protocol for indigestion and are taken alongside meals to decrease acid reflux disorder disease and heartburn. When you enjoy diarrhea, you are given binding treatment; when you experience constipation, you're taking stool softeners. Anti-nausea tablets for nausea and vomiting locate their manner into the drugs cupboard.

These medicinal drugs turn out to be the norm, and after time, you may phrase they become an awful lot a whole lot less powerful, however the factor consequences grow to be increasingly glaring. Over time they are capable of purpose a first-rate deal destruction to our our bodies, main to ulcers, kidney or liver troubles, and usually may motive continual contamination. These capsules reputation on calming the symptoms you're experiencing, however what is the underlying purpose? This critical question dreams addressing.

Your body is particular. It has its specific way of healing itself and maintaining a experience of balance inside the complete body. A disruption inside the norm often results in digestive and GI signs and symptoms, as those referred to above. Something is worrying the body and inflicting this response. When we experience those signs and signs and symptoms and signs and symptoms and symptoms, our first concept is to run to the scientific medical doctor. You are prescribed pills to make your day greater feasible, however you may find yourself returning to the health practitioner all once more. If the ones signs and signs and signs and symptoms return, the medical doctor may endorse similarly research with a specialist and prescribe you the identical set of tablets or perhaps even a better dosage. Let us be honest, how masses of you have got got observed up with a representative or seemed in addition into the inspiration of the troubles being skilled? It can be difficult to control a while in case your venture or finances do now not allow it. It is straightforward to maintain using the ones tablets, which give treatment for a brief period.

You may also additionally turn to diets, exercising, and manner of life fads to assist alleviate the ones signs and symptoms. These equipment can re-energize you and cast off steady fatigue. Alas, they work for a minute, or they do no longer work at all. You may moreover feel barely higher, but it does no longer assist even as there may be little trade physical. The equipment do not constantly artwork because of the fact no longer all diets, exercise, or lifestyles are for you.

Although large pharma also can promote you all types of medicinal capsules that assist, there may be no individual treatment for all things. Since on the identical time as has one-length-fits-all ever labored for honestly all people? It has now not. It may additionally

additionally moreover cover a massive fashion of individuals, however it cannot account for all. The treatment created through the usage of massive pharmaceutical businesses continues people in a loop of returning. These pills provide immediately remedy, which makes us experience higher and capable of waft approximately our day. Every time the ones signs and signs and symptoms flare up all over again, the pills are the primary region we turn to. You can also excursion with those tablets if you have skilled chronic digestive or GI conditions, mainly in case you are out socially for the day. Pleading along with your frame and hoping it holds itself collectively inside the suggest time only works some times. The body has its way of doing topics. Think of those symptoms and studies as greater than tough. Think of it as a be-careful call and a name to interest.

The diets, bodily video video games, and way of life fads promoted are not rooted in fitness on the center. It is generally surface-degree assist and facilities spherical without delay gratification, just like Big Pharma medicinal pills. Your DNA, environment, and food plan play a vital function in how you adapt to these techniques and the manner it affects you. What works for others won't artwork as properly or the least bit for you, that may be a-okay! Don't give up simply however, there are amazing strategies to heal. You in reality should comprehend and recognize your very personal body and artwork with it.

When you recognize and put in force what works exquisite to your frame, you can see the modifications you have got have been given strived in the direction of for years. This is wherein facts the body and body structures are available. Once to procure the get right of entry to code, you could manage your frame right into a enjoy of stability and health irrespective of the environment you're surrounded with the aid of, what's for your DNA, the sort of way of lifestyles you return from, or what everyone has ever said about the ailments or situations you have were given faced. You can trade it all. You can be the saving grace you have were given continuously desired. You honestly wished a amateur's manual. Only you can completely understand your body, how it reacts to positive topics, and the manner it makes you experience. Let this be your initial tool in knowledge what no longer to do to your frame. In doing this, you can short recognize what you may do to permit common health.

You have reached for this book because of the fact a few factor approximately it resonates with you. If most of your uncomfortable symptoms and symptoms are felt within the belly hollow location, you could have concept about your gut. You are surely at the right song! Hippocrates recommended maximum ailments start within the intestine, and he have become no longer an extended way off. Gut contamination is in the back of awful immunity, which permits for an surroundings in the gut that promotes GI dissatisfied and situations related to an infected gut.

Right from the instant you eat, until you release waste within the frame, those techniques all play a feature in intestine health and entire frame, thoughts, and soul wellness. Having guidance on what meals to devour and what the ones meals encompass makes all of the distinction to the intestine. By expertise and knowledge the distinctiveness of your body, you may recognize just what to feed it. This e-book will trade the manner you apprehend your body and its features. The data obtained via this e-book is a manual for the relaxation of your existence. A wholesome and balanced intestine is step one in recuperation your frame and underlying situations you have been unaware of.

You had been residing with ache and pain for some time, and masses of human beings do not even understand it. You also can furthermore have ordinary its presence and determined out to stay with it. Yet, this doesn't make it any less tough. Every day you need to maintain on collectively together with your normal and be mobile irrespective of how masses goes on on your thoughts and intestine. You are genuinely a warrior. Having to combat invisible battles each day and keep a genial facade on the outside can be heavy paintings. Living with an invisible or hidden infection can be putting aside. It can also even have you ever ever doubting your self and what you've got been doing. It can also sense like it is enthusiastic about your head, especially at the identical time as the signs and symptoms are moderate, but your anxiety isn't. Well, intestine inflammation affects your thoughts.

Unfortunately, pretty a few us stay like this with out finding eternal personal consolation. Most days, you preserve it collectively until you may be on your very private private space and decompress from keeping it all collectively. Just each different day, am I proper? Hearing about a brand new manner to assist your symptoms and symptoms and heal your intestine may additionally have you ever rolling your eyes. You probable revel in you have got were given been thru it all and already tried all of the supposedly pinnacle stuff. You can be mentally exhausted and weary, and it is able to seem like every other sadness ready to reveal up. The difference with this ebook is that it shows you the way to paintings together with your unique frame and nature. Two factors are running collectively in harmony as they were doing because the sunrise of time. It genuinely can't fail, but it can take time to locate the satisfactory healthy for you and to start seeing outcomes. As Albert Einstein as quickly as stated, " Problems cannot be solved with the identical mindset that created them." So, preserve trying and preventing for a better tomorrow because you are sturdy enough to prevail.

You will see your frame as more than a smooth vessel but as one with unlocked capacity. Understanding how your thoughts, frame, and soul paintings collectively will help you launch intellectual, bodily, and religious roadblocks. It is laid low with the surroundings you skip in and those you create. Gut infection and terrible health are affected by the beyond and gift. It can be stricken by past scientific clinical doctors who you enjoy may additionally additionally have failed you. Medicine is evolving, and people are relearning the antique and herbal strategies. These strategies were tested for years, increasing sturdiness and preventing continual ailments from progressing.

This e-book holds the blueprint to middle healing. Join others which includes you in rediscovering your body and converting how you have perceived it for years. The body is extra than a vessel; it's miles a dwelling organism and desires your care.

One manner to alleviate irritation inside the thoughts, muscles, and intestine is through freeing stress and movement. Breathing strategies assist loosen tight muscle mass, smooth intellectual fog, and create a non violent and calm surroundings. It aids in calming the intestine by using way of clearing annoying expressions. Breathing strategies are identified to resource the digestion technique as properly. Stress can reason a combat-or-flight response which motives infection. These sports activities may be completed every time and anywhere and let you discover consolation. It's about developing a wholesome environment that benefits your whole health. Here are five breathing techniques called Pranayama (Douillard, 2018). These respiration techniques form a part of Ayurveda practices.

The first exercise requires breathing in through your proper nostril and then exhaling through the left nostril. After that, inhale via your left nose and exhale via your proper nostril. The nostril thru that you final exhaled becomes the nostril through that you inhale. Keep this sample for ten cycles. You may not receive as real with it, however this peculiar and easy workout stimulates the mind and heightens thoughts cognizance.

The second breathing method calls on the way to roll your tongue inwards alongside its period. Your tongue need to resemble a small difficult taco shell. This respiratory technique calls as a manner to inhale through your mouth, maintain that tongue position, and exhale through your nostril. This method cools the body down and distresses the pinnacle and neck on the same time as assisting in pinnacle digestion.

The 1/three exercising calls so you can deliver your teeth collectively as if you are smiling tough. Inhalation is thru the mouth, and exhalation is through the nostril. As you inhale, if you pay hobby a hissing sound, you're doing it right! This approach may additionally have a temper-boosting and cooling impact at the thoughts and body. This respiration technique is idea to purify your senses.

The fourth shape of breathing exercise carries sound power recuperation. Sound energy restoration and vibration are recognized to loosen up the frame. In this breathing technique, you mould your lips to hum. Inhalation and exhalation are via the nostril. Here is the amusing detail! When you exhale, you want to plug out your ears and hum as you breathe out via your nose. This sound resonates through your thoughts and creates a tremendously calming sound. This breathing technique aids in highbrow and emotional well-being.

The fifth workout includes deep breathing with movement. As you stroll spherical, take deep and prolonged breaths in via the nostril, and exhale slowly. These inhalations and exhalations are deep and lengthy in-drawn breath. The equal period and breadth of air need to be taken at the same time as inhaling and exhaling. A way to degree that is to take 5 steps at the same time as breathing in and every different 5 steps even as exhaling. Ten steps may be taken for a extra profound revel in, however most effective when you have the lung capability. This respiratory approach aids in calming and receives your blood pumping.

How do you feel now? Have you discovered a exchange in mood, highbrow clarity, or stomach rest? These clean but intentional respiratory techniques can profoundly effect you and only take approximately ten minutes or a lot less. This is most effective a tease of the comfort you could start to enjoy if you take a look at the outlines of this ebook. You will revel in like a today's person at the aspect of intellectual recovery, wholesome ingesting, and bodily actions. Forget about returning to the vintage you earlier than the brunt of infection; the fashionable you may supersede that.

Balance is at the middle of the whole thing. You do not can buy highly-priced food or device or sign on for programs. It can all be finished in the consolation of your property and in your non-public time. Healing manifestly lets in you to advantage lengthy-lasting results. Try incorporating those devices into your weight-reduction plan for 2 weeks or much less. Next time you want to achieve for a pain killer, look a drop deeper and note what it's far this is hurting. There are hundreds of herbs which may be anti-inflammatory and full of antioxidants that relieve symptoms of inflammation. Herbal teas yield soothing results, which encompass licorice root, ginger, moringa, lavender, and chamomile. Incorporate turmeric into your drink and be aware the changes. To make it tasty, try a 'golden milk' recipe; it's far a outstanding anti-inflammatory. Minerals which include sea salt or volcanic ash, even the use of crystals as filtration can energize your water. Use a herbal cream containing Frankincense, Boswellia, and CBD for muscle aches. Peppermint allows with numerous troubles, which includes nausea, migraines, and achy joints. While making use of these gadgets, lessen out touchy and processed meals. Over those weeks, take a look at how your frame adapts for the better and may heal it. Healing yourself through nature is hundreds higher on your frame and the future health of your organs.

Chapter 12: The Digestive System

You are what you consume. Well, no longer precisely within the maximum literal experience, but terrible consuming can have you ever ever ever feeling at your worst. Your frame survives at the critical nutrients and minerals you provide it with. In such cases, we can be our worst enemies in sabotaging ourselves regarding the food we select out. The meals we consume topics. Food is made of depend, and so are we! Everything we ingest not only plays a function in our frame's healthy (or terrible) functioning, but thru breakdown and absorption, the food we devour turns into part of us. Food is gas, and similar to when setting gasoline on your car, the exceptional makes a difference. As such, the right gasoline is essential for our fitness, too. The meals we consume topics appreciably, however you remember most of all! This is why it's miles crucial to understand the position meals plays in the frame. This way, you could understand what your body desires to enjoy appropriate.

We have touched on the intestine, additionally known as the GI tract, however this workplace paintings part of a more tool referred to as the digestive tool. The digestive system comprises your mouth, throat, esophagus, stomach, small and large intestines, rectum, and anus. The function of this effective device is in its name. It digests all you vicinity into your mouth and breaks down your food for nutrients. Besides digestion, the digestive system's characteristic is mechanical processing, absorption, secretion of acids, water, enzymes, and salts, and putting off waste merchandise. Overall, this tool takes in out of doors materials and distributes them all through your inner systems for proper utilization and circulating nutrients to all of your cells. Poor digestion can frequently reason bloating, dyspepsia, acid reflux disorder sickness, infected belly lining, or even gastroesophageal reflux sickness GERD. The digestive system's function is captivating in controlling digestion and the way correct you experience. Especially in your intestine!

Business in the Front

The digestive position starts offevolved as rapid as you start smacking your lips! The enzymes that spoil down food flood your mouth whilst a tasty cope with touches your tongue. For a few, it could even begin in advance than with those tantalizing aromas of first rate food! Your salivary glands fill your mouth while on the point of consume. Your glands are chargeable for hormone production, so that they should characteristic successfully for correct saliva secretion. Within your saliva are enzymes referred to as amylase, which useful resource digestion with the useful resource of breaking down the complex carbohydrates for your meal. Saliva moreover gives moisture to make sure your food is going down resultseasily. Have you ever compelled your self to swallow at the equal time as you are feeling nausea, dehydration, or in all likelihood, you're definitely now not playing a particular meal? It may moreover revel in like there is sand to your mouth. The sand feeling occurs at the equal time as little saliva floods your mouth; this can purpose horrible digestion as food isn't always broken down effectively inside the mouth. Lucky for you, there are extra salivary glands. Your three number one glands are your parotid glands placed within the the front of each ears, your submandibular glands underneath your jaw, and your sublingual glands underneath the tongue. All those glands make sure your meals is more wet and might slide down after a radical beat down out of your teeth.

Did you understand your tooth shape a part of the digestive feature? Whereas your salivary glands resource inside the chemical breakdown of complicated carbohydrates, your teeth resource within the bodily breakdown. Your enamel, no matter how plenty of them you have got got had been given, play a large characteristic in chomping your food into smaller debris, making it plenty much less tough to digest! The sharp incisors allow for the tearing and gnawing of meals, and your molars on the lower once more are for crushing and grinding into finer textures for swallowing (Health Library, 2023). Teeth fitness is similarly vital, mainly its impact on the microbiome. Just as right consuming and food assets beneficial useful useful resource in a healthy gut, vitamins absorbed with the useful resource of the digestive device useful resource in growing healthful and robust tooth. A healthy eating plan wealthy in fiber, protein, complete grains, veggies, and calcium ensures sturdy tooth and a healthier intestine microbiome. Harmful materials alongside excessively sweet food, carbonated liquids, acidic meals, and difficult sweet can damage enamel tooth and feed the terrible bacteria within the mouth. Damaged enamel enamel can motive enamel decay, and a dysbiosis of bacteria within the mouth can eat away at the teeth, purpose mouth ulcers and go away us with foul-smelling breath. Remember this titbit whilst indulging in sugars a piece too much!

Chapter 13: Micro Biomes Chain Reaction

All about the Microbiota

Did your microbiome is a fruits and cultivation of generations of existence by way of using your predecessors? The specific microorganisms on your intestine immediately stop result from your mom, your grandmother, and the mothers in advance than all of them! Diets at some point of the generations create precise genomes and microorganisms which might be handed down via the genes and diets of the mother, growing the offspring's microbiome. Specific intolerances or sensitivities are because of the microbiome and what it's far aware of the way to cope with. The microbiome can be concept of because of the reality the DNA of health and fitness, the exceptional microbiome make-up creates the genome to fitness, health and contamination. The microbiome's charter is typically in which genetic illnesses display up, however if we trade the weight-reduction plan and join the dysbiosis in the microbiome, we are able to commonly save you the genetic illnesses from arising. The fame quo of the microbiome begins offevolved in utero. The prebiotics and probiotics which are a part of the pregnant mom's weight-reduction plan useful aid in growing the fetus' immune fitness and digestion, giving it the proper nutrients for useful improvement. A mom's microbiome's fitness is important to the toddler's microbiome in utero and after transport.

As the infant passes via the begin canal, they're uncovered to loads of microbes (Stephens, 2023). This first exposure introduces the little one to numerous critical microbes for the immune device. It has been examined that vaginally added toddlers have received microbiota pretty just like maternal vaginal vegetation and are ruled thru the use of Lactobacillus, Prevotella, and Sneathia spp. (Dieterich et al., 2018). Infants added thru Cesarean section (C-section) may be greater at risk of bronchial bronchial bronchial asthma and immune troubles in comparison to babies delivered vaginally because of their lack of exposure to particular microbes. In a C-segment transport, the microbiota that obviously occurs on the pores and pores and skin, e.G., Staphylococcus, Corynebacterium, and Propionibacterium spp., aren't very just like maternal pores and pores and skin microbiota (Dieterich et al., 2018). Infants born via C-segment do not have the critical defensive microbes placed inside the vaginal canal, causing them to be at an advanced hazard of ailment related to immune characteristic, due to issues with the mucosal immune tool (Kristensen jhghj& Henriksen, 2016). Additionally, thru breastfeeding, appropriate intestine micro organism is transferred to the infant, making breastfeeding the number one desire in elevating a wholesome little one.

The type of the microorganisms discovered in prebiotics and probiotics is crucial to the development and fitness of each mother and infant. Exposure to microorganisms will boom your microorganism's range, primary to a stronger immune machine.

The microbiome is home to trillions of microorganisms referred to as the microbiota. Microbes are decided on your pores and pores and skin, inside the mucosa, breathing tract, GI tract (intestine), mammary glands, and the structures associated with your genitals. The most extraordinary microbiome lives within the intestine and mouth due to the mucosal layer. A healthful microbiome is important to a healthy intestine and immunity. The gut is on the center of the health of your entire body. Nutrients are absorbed and unfold to the relaxation of the frame thru the intestine. These nutrients are critical for the features of your frame systems, which includes the immune systems, endocrine structures, lymphatic systems, and proper cognitive capabilities. The microbiome and plenty of microorganisms in the gut play a great feature in protective your frame from infections and ailments via the use of speakme with the immune cells. The human microbiota consists of of 10-one hundred trillion symbiotic microbial cells harbored with the useful resource of anybody, frequently within the form of bacteria in the gut. The intestine is covered with each proper and horrific micro organism. An imbalance of the microbiome and flowers of the intestine may additionally result in GI disillusioned, unpleasant bodily signs, and chronic illnesses.

Microorganisms of the gut are various, which includes bacteria, viruses, and fungi. The extra the microorganism range and variety, the more fitness you can revel in because of the truth exquisite microorganisms play incredible roles. The extra strains of microorganisms your frame is exposed to, the better your microbiome's capability to react to every of these strains before they may harm you.

Microorganisms' variety is finished thru a numerous weight loss plan and exposure to many environments. We should apprehend micro organism as neither top nor awful however as an alternative by how our our our our bodies react to an appropriate bacteria. A healthful microbiome can discover the presence of in all likelihood dangerous micro organism and will act due to this. Consequently, your immune system will become higher ready to conquer future harmful bacteria and viral ailments. If we do now not have a properly-flourishing microbiome, the dangerous micro organism will populate and overtake the excellent strains of bacteria in the intestine.

Microorganisms are all spherical you and might locate their manner into your body like germs, so we're taught to live hygienic. Microorganisms aren't all lousy; some resource in making you stronger and extra healthy. By being over-hygienic, we emerge as killing the good bacteria, too, leaving us with plenty plenty much less of a severa microbiome. The microorganisms of your microbiome need to be in symbiosis, so our hobby is to find out the stableness and maintain it as splendid as viable.

Foods and dietary supplements that characteristic prebiotics, probiotics, and digestible fibers feed and growth the many unique microorganisms. The genetic range inside our gut microbiota permits us to digest compounds thru metabolic pathways not explicitly coded for within the mammalian genome, notably developing our capability to extract electricity from our numerous diets (Ursell et al., 2012).

The genetic range of microorganisms within your intestine is liable for how your body digests, absorbs, reabsorbs, and dispatches essential nutrients, minerals, and nutrients. Due to gene sequencing, a malformation of a gene and protein, or a horrible weight loss plan, some people can also have an entire lot a whole lot much less microorganism variety important to an imbalance in gut fitness. Microorganisms' range is more first-rate through dietary inclusions.

A food regimen rich in prebiotics and probiotics from severa assets will increase the lines of microorganisms inside the gut. The exposition to new and numerous components introduces the gut to numerous new microorganisms. Not continuously will one be able to cope with the ones new ingredients in case you do no longer have the appropriate microbiome had to digest these materials. Starting slowly and eating them constantly in small portions might also add some discomfort initially. However, once you have got the right microbiome to cope with the meals, your gut will start to gain from their many blessings. Using a medical doctor or train well suggested in this area is essential to ensure no underlying issues are causing the pain from those components. Someone stricken by SIBO will first need to remove fibers given that there may be an overgrowth, and once they smooth the underlying trouble, they could begin such as again in the pre and probiotics to build up their advantages. Microbes can considerably boom the type of metabolic system of the human intestine, permitting you to digest an array of substrates (Ursell et al., 2012). A form of microorganisms outcomes in less difficult digestion of various materials and allows your frame systems to function correctly. A healthy, various, and balanced microbiome aids in a sturdy immune tool and lends to a sturdy GI barrier function. Change does no longer continuously come clean however the reward is always more making it a well surely well worth struggle.

The GI barrier talents as a wall that filters thru nutrients, minerals, vitamins, and water from the small intestines to vital systems in the frame. This wall is in component permeable, so the frame absorbs critical products, and pollutants and waste are washed out. A balanced gut microbiome allows for the proper digestion and absorption of vitamins. A "middle microbiome includes the maximum widespread phylotypes and is hypothesized to hold the realistic stability and homeostasis crucial for a healthful environment" (Riedel et al., 2014).

An imbalanced gut is a microbiome in dysbiosis. When this takes place, the gut's barrier feature also can come to be too permeable because of developing quantities of risky gut micro organism within the small gut. When the barrier wall is being eaten away due to the inhospitable environment, best gut micro organism, which protects the gut, is overpowered. A horrible GI barrier lets in dangerous bacteria, pollutants, and waste to flow into the bloodstream with the crucial vitamins, minerals, nutrients, and water. This is referred to as leaky intestine syndrome. Leaky intestine syndrome may moreover bring about excessive GI conditions which include Crohn's sickness, IBD, Celiac disorder, and polycystic ovarian syndrome (PCOS). A balanced microbiome is crucial in strengthening the GI barrier characteristic for the reason that it is wherein critical digestion and reabsorption take place, fueling the frame's device and balancing it.

The gut microbiome impacts your frame's herbal immune device. The vitamins absorbed contribute to the nicely-being of the immune device. A healthful immune gadget is an indication of a healthful intestine. A terrible intestine is accompanied through the usage of low immunity and concurrent infection. Inflammation in the body is because of risky micro organism, infections, viruses, and particles decided as threatening for your immune system. Gut dysbiosis motives irritation, and your immune tool dispatches inflammatory cells to heal the frame and combat off infections. When this takes location for prolonged intervals, the immune machine might also moreover get pressured and function exquisite responses. The immune cells start attacking the healthy cells of the GI tract. Stiffness and tingling in any limbs, arms, and toes is a not unusual issue impact. This might also moreover bring about further infection inside the shape of bowel inflammation, along with IBS or IBD. This everyday infection, lousy intestine health, and coffee immunity similarly ruin your gut. This may moreover leave you liable to a bunch of GI conditions and diseases, which include Crohn's sickness, ulcerative colitis, and colon cancers.

As a cease end result of this inflammation within the gut, the mucosal layer that lines and strengthens the GI tract turns into thinner and plenty less effective. The developing quantity of risky bacteria diminishes the epithelial cells of the mucosal lining. The sticky substance secreted via the use of the mucosa is a protecting and preventive measure from the fluids that shape a part of digestion within the GI tract. A bad and inflamed mucosa layer results in intestinal permeability and damages the stomach's lining. The mucosal layers of the stomach shield the lining from becoming inflamed and eroding due to the strong pH of gastric fluids. Damage to the mucosal layer within the belly due to an inflamed gut permits for an increasingly more acidic surroundings within the stomach that destroys the stomach lining. This effects in peptic (gastric) ulcers. A balanced intestine microbiome is crucial for a healthful mucosa that protects the frame and creates an surroundings for self-repair. The mucosal layer traces the digestive and GI tract from the mouth to the anus. A faulty or minimized mucosa may additionally depart the whole body unprotected and susceptible. Aloe vera is proven to help soothe the mucosal lining at the issue of strengthening tissue and can be beneficial in recovery the intestine.

How do you gain intestine dysbiosis, you could wonder? It is in preferred a give up result of negative eating regimen and unbalanced eating. It can also come approximately from parasites or mildew we're available in contact with which might be left untreated. A restrictive weight loss plan, further to meals with fewer prebiotics and probiotics, ends in a far plenty much less various microbiome. A diet plan deficient in fibers, minerals, and vitamins leads to intestine dysbiosis and a terrible immune system. Most diets are complete of sensitive sugars, subtle carbohydrates, and fatty elements that don't feed the coolest gut microbiome however the horrific. If you are not consuming fibers to feed the amazing gut microbiome, ingesting to create gut symbiosis, or ingesting numerous elements, you are allowing the dangerous bacteria to multiply. This results in GI dissatisfied, which develops into conditions of the GI tract. Your gut desires an entire lot of microorganisms and live cultures from meals that boom the wide sort of microorganisms and functions thereof within the microbiome. The large this range, the much less possibly intestine dysbiosis takes place. Certainly, now not even as your proper intestine bacteria within the microbiome are having a banquet!

Impacts of an Imbalanced Microbiome

An unbalanced gut microbiome outcomes in dysbiosis inside the GI tract and the organs and structures surrounding it. If the feature of the intestine is horrible because of infection, how can your frame acquire all the goodness it desires for effective functioning? Simply talking, it does not. PCOS is known as a end result of intestinal permeability because of terrible intestine health. Nutrient deficiencies, insulin resistance, and inflammation within the reproductive vicinity accompany PCOS.

Often, this syndrome may additionally cause dysmenorrhea or amenorrhea that affects fertility. Dysmenorrhea is painful durations and immoderate prostaglandins because of a hormonal imbalance. Amenorrhea is at the same time as humans leave out their intervals for months on quit, or they now not get preserve of it, that would all be related to hormonal imbalance and inflammation. Gut dysbiosis and infection are linked to hormonal imbalances. Your microbes produce an enzyme referred to as beta-glucuronidase that converts estrogen into its lively paperwork. A dysbiosis within the microbiome can purpose an imbalance of estrogen. Gut contamination is likewise related to stomach and pelvic contamination. A intestine not effectively soaking up and freeing important vitamins into the frame outcomes in structures and abilities turning into nutrient terrible. PCOS is connected to magnesium, diet D, B vitamins, and folate deficiencies. These deficiencies and hormonal imbalances have an impact on ovary feature and development, thyroid, estrogen, progesterone, and androgen levels. These nutrients are observed in prebiotic and probiotic components. When you aren't giving your body those meals or if the kingdom of your intestine is struggling to digest these food because of contamination, those nutrient deficiencies can also moreover furthermore upward thrust up.

Dysbiosis and contamination in the gut have an effect on liver characteristic. The liver is accountable for excreting pollution and waste products from the body, together with ridding extra hormones. Excess hormones no longer filtered out can also moreover result in toxin assemble-up and in addition hormonal imbalance, resulting in estrogen dominance within the frame and once in a while too little estrogen. Excess hormones within the body may also prevent ovulation. Not most effective that, however you could enjoy pelvic infection or ache, gastric reflux, and nausea. A terrible, inflamed intestine microbiome results in vain liver feature. A leaky intestine leaks pollution and waste, sowing discord in the bloodstream and the reproductive tract, vital to toxin build-up and inflammatory responses.

Inflammation of the microbiome may additionally have an effect at the mind, too. The gut-mind axis (GBA) is the connection the microbiome has with the thoughts. What you eat and the way your frame reacts right away have an effect on the thoughts. These outcomes are every cognitive and mental. What goes on inside the intestine affects the vitamins and messages sent to the thoughts. The ache and consequences of GI disappointed cause tension and pressure, affecting highbrow and social health. As you are starting to see, intestine health affects the whole body extra than the physical.

A poor diet does now not make a contribution to healthy cognition. Inflammation of the intestine ends in inflammation inside the thoughts. A intestine that isn't wholesome, balanced, or rife with suitable micro organism is visible thru belief approaches, styles, and highbrow skills due to the reality irritation in the gut may impair rapid concept techniques. The enteric anxious machine (ENS) works with the large worried system (CNS) to create the intestine-thoughts axis, which serves as a hyperlink maximum of the "emotional and cognitive facilities of the brain with peripheral intestinal skills" (Carabotti et al., 2015).

The ENS uses the vagus nerve due to the fact the medium of communique most of the intestine and the thoughts. The ENS is the mini mind that sends signs and symptoms in your thoughts. "This interplay amongst microbiota and GBA appears to be bidirectional, mainly via signaling from intestine-microbiota to mind and from thoughts to intestine-microbiota via neural, endocrine, immune, and humoral links" (Carabotti et al., 2015). Myelination is the formation of myelin sheath determined on neuron cells, which allows provide the inspiration for mind connectivity. Dysbiosis inside the microbiome can skew the creation of myelination, unfavourable neuron cells and causing neurological damage. The vagus nerve is one of the twelve cranial nerves that run from the lower prevent of the mind to the big intestines—the vagus nerve branches into 3 openings One being the throat, two being the backbone and ears, and 3 being the lungs, coronary heart, and esophagus. The vagus nerve has the ability to save you food from engaging in digestion and plays a vital role in health.

Chapter 14: Complications Inside The Digestive Tract

Poor Gut Health and Physical Illness

Digestive troubles relate to situations of the digestive tract which have an impact on you each day. Digestive problems can start off as moderate symptoms collectively with nausea and belly ache, however if left to worsen, they are able to grow to be continual ailments over the years. It can have an impact on extra than genuinely your bodily self; it could have an effect in your highbrow fitness as nicely. Individuals who be troubled by manner of persistent digestive issues undergo on a persistent daily basis, with the more stress and strain of fluctuating signs and symptoms and symptoms and signs (Greber, 2018). Living with ailments that bring about awful digestion is physical, mentally, and emotionally draining. If you've got decided on to study in addition in this book, you have possibly professional this toll. I clearly have, too, and some days may be tough! There are many situations associated with complications within the digestive tract, and what is worse is you can boom more than the form of conditions. The root of a majority of these conditions lies within the intestine, so we need to no longer recognition at the labels we are given however as an possibility art work on solving the underlying purpose of all of it.

If issues rise up inside the course of digestion, this can considerably offset the stability of bacteria within the intestine. Indigestion happens because of terrible consuming behavior that don't align together with your genetic composition. Certain components you're ingesting can be an contamination on your particular microbiota. If you are not ingesting consistent with your dosha, ingesting too speedy or too much, and consuming at improper hours of the day, this may all make contributions to indigestion. Common food contributing to indigestion encompass fried food, trans fatty additives, copious portions of caffeine and caffeinated beverages, excessive in sugar and carbonated beverages, and ingesting too many touchy sugars. These food picks can result in dyspepsia, heartburn, stomachaches, nausea, and esophageal pain. These inflammatory responses cease stop result from horrible digestion and contribute to an imbalance of intestine microorganisms. The response of your intestine to those meals relies upon on your genetic makeup and the chemical composition of your GI tract.

An imbalance of microorganisms within the intestine is referred to as dysbiosis. The imbalance of microorganisms within the gut can be due to micro organism, fungal infections, or parasites (Greber, 2018). Remember how most of the digestion and absorption of vital nutrients occurs on this area? Well, simply do not forget the variety of nutrients misplaced and the ache that arises internal an inhospitable environment within the intestine. The intestine microbiome consists of appropriate gut microorganisms and horrible gut microorganisms. Harmful meals contributing to bad gut bacteria are processed food, excessively consuming hard cheeses, excessive caffeine, sugars, and synthetic sweeteners. What your gut desires is a severa and colorful diet. To increase the best gut micro organism and promote microorganism stability for your gut, you have to study ingesting fresher meals, incorporating home-cooked food, eating fiber, and lots much less delicate carbohydrates.

Additionally, you need to encompass probiotic nutritional nutritional supplements and rent fermented meals which includes kimchi, sauerkraut, yogurt, and kefir; my preferred being kombucha. These materials beneficial useful resource in proper digestion. A wholesome dietary stability creates appropriate gut health (Greber, 2018). A healthful diet plan does no longer advise you need to be on a strict vegetable diet or save you playing some aspect that offers you a burst of serotonin.

www.ingramcontent.com/pod-product-compliance
Lightning Source LLC
Chambersburg PA
CBHW062140020426
42335CB00013B/1281